Mom's OK,
She Just Forgets

Mom's OK, She Just Forgets

The Alzheimer's Journey
from Denial to Acceptance

Evelyn McLay and
Ellen P. Young

Forewords by Barry Gordon, MD, PhD, and
Henry Weinberg, PhD

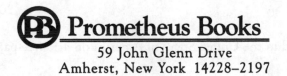

Prometheus Books

59 John Glenn Drive
Amherst, New York 14228–2197

Published 2007 by Prometheus Books

Inquiries should be addressed to
Prometheus Books
59 John Glenn Drive
Amherst, New York 14228-2197
VOICE: 716-691-0133, ext. 207
FAX: 716-564-2711
WWW.PROMETHEUSBOOKS.COM

11 10 09 08 07   5 4 3 2 1

Library of Congress Cataloging-in-Publication Data

McLay, Evelyn D.
   Mom's ok, she just forgets : the Alzheimer's journey from denial to acceptance / by Evelyn D. McLay and Ellen P. Young ; foreword by Barry Gordon ; foreword by Henry Weinberg.
       p. cm.
   Includes bibliographical references.
   ISBN 13: 978-1-59102-469-9 (pbk : alk. paper)
   ISBN 10: 1-59102-469-2 (pbk : alk. paper)
   1. Alzheimer's disease. 2. Alzheimer's disease—Patients—Care.
3. Alzheimer's disease—Patients—Family relationships. 4. Alzheimer's disease—Social aspects. I. Young, Ellen P. II. Title.

RC523.M41 2007
616.8'31—dc22   2006022443

Printed in the United States of America on acid-free paper

*All vignettes, scenarios, and
examples used in this book
are both true and anonymous.
They reflect a blend of personal and
clinical experiences of both authors.*

Contents

Acknowledgments

We are so very grateful to all of the following people. Each one has made a substantial or significant contribution to bringing this book to fruition. Thank you to the wonderful people who work at the Greater Maryland Chapter of the Alzheimer's Association: especially Cass Naugle, Shelley Northern Jennings, Lisa Brakebill, and Diane Wit. At Prometheus Books: Steven L. Mitchell, editor in chief, Jean Andrzejewski, and all of the editors, artists, production, marketing, and promotional people—you have all been great. Thanks to Hirsh Goldberg, our literary agent, who has always supported this project, and to Marie Ichrath, who helped Evelyn out of her denial. Thank you to Barry Gordon, MD, PhD, and Henry Weinberg, PhD, for writing such wonderful forewords. Also, to our friends and willing "readers," Charles Calvert, Sylvia Hildner, Ann Keene, and Sr. Genevieve Kunkel. Thank you to Mary Faith Ferretto, Allan Anderson, MD, and Jean Tucker Mann.

Our families, who know our hearts, also deserve much gratitude. Thanks to Bruce McLay for countless hours on the computer and for his love and support, and to Jonathan Tung, who always lends his support and love. Thanks to Wayne Verity (for all the help with the computer), Lynne Flynn, and their spouses, Robin and Michael, for loving support once again.

Foreword

An individual's family and friends are often in a far better position than healthcare professionals to appreciate changes in memory, judgment, and personality—in short, the features of dementing conditions such as Alzheimer's disease. With this special knowledge comes a special responsibility. When do the memory lapses and errors in judgment become the rule, rather than the exception? When do they cease being irritations and exasperations, but instead become harbingers of a dread disease? How can different members of a family—with different perspectives, hopes, fears, and knowledge—agree on each of the painful decisions that need to be made, even when they often agree on nothing at all?

Mom's OK, She Just Forgets offers a perspective on these realizations and decisions that has not been given the attention it deserves, despite the large body of literature for families about Alzheimer's disease. The book's authors discuss some of the earliest—as well as the most challenging—situations and behaviors with a breadth of understanding, an attention to detail, and a compassion for all involved that is unusual in the field.

While family and friends bear the initial burden of deciding whether something is seriously wrong with their loved one, qualified healthcare professionals must still evaluate all the evidence about an individual and weigh it against all the possibilities, before arriving at a provisional, or a more certain, diagnosis. Families and friends should not feel that the diagnostic burden is theirs; it is not.

But it is, of course, family and friends—not clinicians—who have to live with newly diagnosed individuals. It is for them that *Mom's OK, She Just Forgets* will resonate most strongly and provide the most valuable insights. The authors draw on both their own experience and that of many others.

Because they have been there already, they illuminate the challenging road ahead.

Barry Gordon, MD, PhD
Professor of Neurology and Cognitive Science
Founder, The Memory Clinic
The Johns Hopkins Medical Institutions
Baltimore, Maryland

Foreword

Life can sometimes throw us off balance. We may have achieved a satisfactory status quo, an organization of our relationships with others and the world in general, and then something happens. We are faced with an event that is unexpected and for which we are unprepared, a loss of a significant part of the structure we have developed and on which we depend. Despite the discomfort and even pain of the experience, most of us resort to the tools that have helped us in the past to cope with this present upheaval and work toward a new set of adaptations.

Thinking in terms of "loss" may be helpful in understanding the impact of Alzheimer's disease. It can be viewed as a loss, not only by the person with Alzheimer's, in terms of cognition and physical capabilities, but also by those who are in psychologically significant relationships with this person. These may or may not be family members who ultimately provide the caregiving. It is with these caregivers that this book is primarily concerned, with a very practical, down-to-earth approach.

As psychologists, we are familiar with the vast body of literature over the past decades dealing with loss and the adaptation to it. The loss may be sudden, as in time of war, or the result of natural catastrophe, or it may be drawn out, as in the case of terminal illness or even the loss of a physical capacity. In all of these situations, the survivor must recognize the loss, and over time, work out a new set of adaptations. Some of us, for one reason or another, cannot immediately accept the loss; but over time, bit by bit, we are able to do the reworking. Time alone does not do the healing, but gives us the opportunity to work at it. We also have found that there is a small group of individuals who cannot recognize or accept loss at all but instead react to any change as a catastrophic threat. Their psychological fragility or lack of resilience may, instead, lead to physical symptoms or even self-destructive behavior. Thus "denial," in its many forms, a theme running through this book, may be an adaptive coping technique when used by most of us to buy more time to deal actively with the loss. However, it may be maladaptive when the reality of loss is completely shut out, as in the extreme example just described.

Complicating the response to Alzheimer's disease is an insidious set of opportunities for denial, first on the part of the sufferer who may deny and confabulate in minimizing the cognitive losses, and on the part of the caregiver, who can't keep up with the destabilizing changes presented by the sufferer. The caregiver, like the person with Alzheimer's, may also try to minimize or at least slow down the recognition and acceptance of reality. Alzheimer's may also signify losses for the caregiver that are more difficult than other types to accept, since "the person" is still there, yet not there. The ambiguities often result in frustrated expectations and, in many cases, anger followed by guilt over such feelings.

Mom's Ok, She Just Forgets deals more with the caregivers' side of the relationship. Using their own personal experiences as caregivers, and also as counselors of other caregivers, the authors have provided a sensitive, empathic approach to the needs of those who find themselves in this situation. They provide an opportunity for caregivers to realize that what they may feel to be unique (and sometimes even "bad") may really not be unique but, in fact, be felt by other caregivers. Also, they make clear the fact that it is normal for caregivers to feel a sense of personal inadequacy in meeting the new demands. The authors apply their obviously hard-earned wisdom to help further the adequate coping of those who come after. My own assessment is that just picking up this most readable book will be a major first step in benefiting from what the authors have to offer.

Henry Weinberg, PhD
Professor Emeritus
Boston University
Boston, Massachusetts

Introduction

**Hope is the thing with feathers
That perches in the soul. . . .**

—Emily Dickinson

This is a book about Alzheimer's disease (AD). It is different from any other book on the subject in that it strongly emphasizes the issue of "denial." Denial is the most pervasive coping mechanism. We can all succumb to its beguiling relief. However, within the realm of Alzheimer's, denial can, and sometimes does, behave like an ever-present albatross that hovers over caregivers and their loved ones with dementia. It becomes infused into many of the issues and problems that they face, from diagnosis throughout the entire journey.

Denial, not worked through, becomes our enemy when we are dealing with Alzheimer's disease. With no cure and nothing on the horizon, it may seem to be an acceptable approach. However, currently there are effective medications that might inhibit the disease process. Early diagnosis is crucial because, while the progress of the disease is held back, a vaccine or improved medications could be developed. Moreover, early diagnosis facilitates proper care and management of loved ones with dementia. It allows for important medical, financial, and legal issues to be given prompt attention. Denial can thwart sensible and needed action all along the painful Alzheimer's journey.

The human mind is mysterious. Each of the secrets medical science uncovers seems to reveal still more mystery. One thing is certain: our psyches are well protected, with denial at the top of the list of our ego defenses.

Recognition of denial and understanding its negative aspects can help caregivers feel more in control and put them in a more positive frame of mind. Our efforts in this book will focus on all the obstacles confronting caregivers on the labyrinthine path with their loved ones. We gently direct them, with signposts along the way, to paths of action that lead to healing the wounded spirit. And we hope that, eventually, those paths lead caregivers to make progress, one small step at a time, toward acceptance of a devastating diagnosis and all that goes with it.

To even think about a diagnosis of Alzheimer's or any irreversible form of dementia strikes fear in our hearts. Most people would rather put their heads in the sand and use any of the many psychological defense mechanisms—especially denial—to avoid thinking about it. One of the more obvious ways denial works its way into our psyches is dealing with "the driving dilemma." We often say and do everything we can to postpone dealing with the issue indefinitely. A loved one with Alzheimer's can be in danger and put others in danger by being behind the wheel of a car. This is just one example of the many manifestations of denial. It also shows how easy it is to unwittingly allow a situation to become dangerous for us and/or our loved one. Denial can wreak havoc with entire families when one member succumbs to Alzheimer's.

Whether it is a broken leg, diabetes, or Alzheimer's disease, a person with an illness is first and foremost a person whose dignity must be honored. That is why we rarely use the word *patient*. We will refer, instead, to *persons with Alzheimer's, persons with dementia, our family member,* or *our loved one.* Alzheimer's disease will sometimes be referred to as *AD, confusion,* or *dementia.* We try to use examples involving both genders equally throughout the book. In reality, however, more women than men are diagnosed with Alzheimer's. The reason is unclear, but the fact that women outlive men by a number of years may be the cause, or at least part of it. Hence our title, *Mom's OK.* Obviously it could be Dad, Husband, Wife— any member of a family.

We authors have both "walked our talk." Evelyn lost her husband, mother-in-law, and sister-in-law to Alzheimer's. Ellen lost her mother and aunt.

Evelyn spent ten years as a support-group facilitator and is currently starting her fifteenth year as a Helpline counselor at the Greater Maryland

Chapter of the Alzheimer's Association. Ellen spent the last fifteen years of a career in social work in a clinical setting at a Baltimore hospital. She retired in 1997 to enjoy her grandchildren and to promote her first book, *Between Two Worlds: Special Moments of Alzheimer's and Dementia* (Prometheus Books, 1999). It is primarily about the healing power of humor.

We believe that our most important task is to share our collective experience with the reader. Though we have different career backgrounds and had different experiences with each of our loved ones with Alzheimer's, we still share many common threads. We hope that, in sharing our collective knowledge and experience, we will become a "lifeline for caregivers." We want to be comforting companions to caregivers. We want to enable them to gradually work through denial and approach their loved ones with a positive attitude and "love in action."

In essence, this book is not clinical, but we believe we have an obligation to present the truth as it now stands with regard to statistics and AD. Roughly 50 percent of people reaching eighty-five years of age are at risk to develop Alzheimer's disease. Though a daunting statistic, it is a reality. We can play ostrich, but the medical evidence is overwhelming. It is pointless to feed our denial. It is far more constructive to pull our heads out of the sand; to be grateful for every waking, thinking moment; and to become advocates for finding a vaccine and/or a cure.

One of the reasons we flee into denial is to block the fear that we, ourselves, might become victims of Alzheimer's someday. We caregivers must begin our own work at avoiding it. Social graces and self-awareness play a significant role in keeping it from becoming apparent. No one can be complacent and say, "It will never happen to me."

A week doesn't go by without some new tip emerging on ways to exercise our brain, usually involving mind-stimulating activities. Physical exercise, good eating habits, vitamins, and socializing are behaviors that are also recommended. We authors feel, while those things are positive, that the message can be misunderstood. The most highly educated, keenest, and sharpest of minds can succumb. We need no reminders of the fact that Alzheimer's is an equal opportunity invader—from presidents to paupers.

There is no cure for AD. There is no avoidance of death. We have no choice in the reality either of loss or of suffering; but we do have a choice in how much we allow ourselves to be crushed by that suffering. Death is as much a part of life as is birth. American culture is collectively in denial. It is a culture of "youth, beauty, and prosperity," and little or no thought is given to reality. When it comes to AD, the reality is we need to find a way to postpone or cure it. Dealing with it is difficult, and finding a cure or vaccine has been elusive. Research continues, and new approaches and medicines to delay the onset are always in the works.

As this book's chapters unfold, many examples of denial are discussed. Driving a vehicle is not the only station along the Alzheimer's journey where denial stops us. Daycare is another. Often, sending a loved one to a daycare program is the answer to many problems encountered when caring for a confused loved one at home. This is especially true if the caregiver works. In chapter 8, the excuses we make to ourselves for not sending our loved one to adult daycare are listed. Caregivers sometimes have a similar, but more profound reaction to the idea of long-term care placement, i.e., nursing homes. They have multiple reasons and excuses as to why they refuse even to explore this avenue.

This book offers practical help and advice, with heartfelt warmth and understanding from two people who have been there. We suggest various behaviors, tools, and techniques for moving beyond denial. Real people who have faced the many problems brought on by AD speak out, with hope, from the pages. They share their journeys from denial to action to an improved attitude, and on to acceptance of their personal plights.

We offer "caregiver relief" by allowing readers to identify with the people in the stories, helping them realize that they are not alone. Caregivers are assured that there are no "bad" caregivers on the Alzheimer's journey. People are where they are for a reason. Self-understanding and acceptance will come about gradually, as proven methods of dealing with problems light the way for readers and gently nudge them forward. Readers will be encouraged. It is helpful to learn about "attitude tune-up," positive actions, and how to keep our sense of humor. There are constant reminders of the need for "patience, perspective, and humor."

Our mantra, which we hope caregivers will repeat to themselves often, is: *I can't be a good caregiver unless I take care of myself.* Basically anything we do in life must begin with ourselves. And that is especially true in providing care for a loved one. If we are tired, upset, sad, or grouchy, people with dementing illnesses will pick up on it. It is as if they have antennae. A smile and a sense of humor are gifts that keep on giving. We can make much more progress when we project that positive attitude. It is important to try, even when we are not in the mood. A smile changes our blood chemistry. So fake it 'til you make it!

We are not making light of the difficulties ahead for the Alzheimer's family. Your loved one has received a devastating diagnosis. But it is you, the reader and caregiver, who must ultimately accept personal responsibility for how positive the atmosphere is for your loved one. The proactive factor always starts with you.

Our hope is that caregivers who read this book and put the information they gain to the test will find themselves moving forward, no matter how bumpy and winding the road may be. It is not an easy journey, and we will not attempt to convince anyone otherwise. But there is always a certain satisfaction gained by mustering up the courage to give our best shot at overcoming adversity and to deal with the problems we encounter in life, no matter how monumental they may be. We authors have been down many of those roads and have had to make our own attitude adjustments along the way. Our plan is to accompany you on your own journey, with map in hand, to provide you with as much needed information as possible.

There are many suggestions for avoiding caregiver burnout between the covers of this book. Chapters 4 and 9 deal specifically with caring for the caregiver. It is encouraging to know that as we move out of denial, we change viewpoints and attitudes. Thus, we change behaviors. All these changes make for more effective and efficient caregiving as we deal with issues such as challenging and aggressive behaviors, difficulty with communication, the need for daycare, and even the need for placement.

We mentioned driving, daycare, and nursing home placement, but we can't say too often that denial enters into every aspect of dealing with Alzheimer's. The chapter format of *Mom's Ok, She Just Forgets* is designed to approach the problems in a manner that is as caregiver-friendly as possible. We hope it rewards you for your courage as you read on and apply some of our suggestions. Actually we hope the book becomes dog-eared, underlined, and wrinkled—a sign that it has become part of the family.

We really do want to share our experiences and hard-won expertise in dealing with Alzheimer's disease. We had to pry open our own hearts as we trod our own difficult roads. We know how important it is to keep feelings, no matter how painful, at a conscious level in order to deal with problems; shutting down, turning off, and tuning out exacts a price from the caregiver, the loved one, and the whole family.

We all have a belief system. Whether we are believers or nonbelievers, we all have spirits. In fact, some say we are spirits having a human experience, not vice versa. Whatever the facts, we need to try to keep our spirits up as we go about our caregiving duties, day after tiring day.

The Alzheimer's journey is a journey of the spirit, for both caregiver and care-receiver. We learn about "the moment" in a new way. The fact that the moment is all we have and all we may ever have is highlighted by this disease. We are wise if we learn to live in the moment and to not be numb to it. While it is tempting to tune out, we do not benefit by allowing our experience with our loved one with AD to become one big blackout—a time when we move and breathe, but do not really live. Everything in this book will lead the caregiver to a place that will refresh his or her ability to live. Things will be "different." We may never quite return to that place we now call "normal." Our loved ones with AD will be living in a reality different from ours. Their sense of time may be lost. The moment is all they have. We hope to guide you in doing your very best to make that moment positive and beautiful.

This is our wish list for our readers (we are positive thinkers and we have BIG WISHES):

- We want this book to be a comforting companion for caregivers.
- We want caregivers to find their way out of denial through love in action.
- We want caregivers to learn a new approach; one that will bring success in dealing with the problems of Alzheimer's disease.
- We want caregivers to flavor their approach with love—both gentle and tough.
- We want caregivers to move into the realm of healing acceptance.
- We want caregivers to be able to accomplish all of the above without losing their sense of humor or their perspective.

Carpe diem. Seize the day.
Let's get to work.

Chapter One

"We Peel the Onion"
Layers of Denial

**Life is like an onion; you peel off one layer at a time,
and sometimes you weep.
—Carl Sandburg**

WHAT IS DENIAL?

Denial is the most important defense mechanism the body employs to shield itself from innumerable situations, from the inconsequential to those that are absolutely life shattering. When faced with the death of a child, the loss of a job, the breakup of a marriage, or Alzheimer's disease, denial becomes an appropriate segment of the grief process. Healthy denial protects the body from initial shock. It acts as insulation until the mind is able to gradually assimilate the catastrophic event. Our natural instincts are at work. We can survive.

Webster defines *denial* as the act of saying no, a refusal to believe or to accept. This definition neatly parallels the response to unwelcome, unwanted, devastating events: "Oh, no, this can't be happening!" "Tell me it is not true!" "I don't want to believe it!" "I cannot believe it!"

This is not an unreasonable response to the suspicion of, or the diagnosis of, Alzheimer's disease. We are reluctant to face the disease that will rob our loved one of his or her cognitive skills. This is a disease that will change our lives in ways we are afraid to contemplate. We think, "Maybe it isn't Alzheimer's disease." Denial becomes our comforter.

We fear the unknown, the black uncertainty of the disease that attacks the brain, the center of what we do and who we are. We, of course, are afraid of ourselves—another unknown. How will we face the challenges of the disease? Will we have the courage, the strength, and the patience to deal with the continuing and changing problems the disease brings to a family? With this disease come changes we have not chosen and do not want.

Denial becomes the comfortable covering that shields our conscious mind from the undesirable, the unacceptable. It soon becomes the effective barrier between us and this unwelcome illness, this unbidden sorrow.

We may think, "We are not in denial. We know Dad has dementia. But it's not that bad. We don't have to do anything now. Maybe later, but not now!"

This is classic avoidance, denial's twin, fed by fear.

Unless we can work our way through denial, it becomes our enemy.

Denial entraps us. It keeps us from seeking information about the disease, keeps us from seeking a professional diagnosis and evaluation. Denial keeps us from obtaining much-needed legal and financial advice. It also prevents us from objectively assessing the cognitive decline in our loved one. Is Mother still able to live alone, or are we placing her in a high-risk situation? Would Dad benefit from the social interaction he would experience in daycare? Is Dad a safe driver? (All these things are discussed in later chapters.)

Denial, in some form, is a problem for every member of an Alzheimer's family. We are not alone.

In this book we hope to provide you, the reader, and your family, the towrope of action and the proper attitude to pull you out of denial. We cannot change the diagnosis, but we can suggest healthy, coping mechanisms and positive attitudes that will banish some of your fears as you "stare the monster down." (In her book *Between Two Worlds*, Ellen gives good examples of people who have been able to do just that.)

DENIAL AS A RESPONSE TO AD

It is important that we tell you up front that denial associated with AD is similar to the many-layered onion. We peel one layer off only to be faced with still another. We face the diagnosis and accomplish all the necessary actions, only to find ourselves in continuing layers of denial:

- "Mom's not ready for daycare."
- "Dad can still drive, can't he?"
- "A support group? Not me!"
- "Nursing home placement? Never!"

Every time there are significant changes in our loved one's behavior, every time these changes impact the comfort, security, and well-being we try so hard to create in the midst of this terrible disease, we become unsettled and disturbed. We have to do *it* again.

What is *it*?

Change, adapt, accept. We have to change our expectations. We have to change our patterns of behavior to adapt to each new stage of the disease:

- "It *is* time for daycare."
- "Dad *cannot* drive anymore."
- "We *need* a support group."
- "*Yes*, a healthcare center is the *best choice* for our loved one."

DENIAL ENTRAPS US

Denial can get as strong a hold on us during the course of the disease as it did in the beginning stages of diagnosis. Denial, the beguiling but harmful comforter, can overtake even the most resolute caregiver.

We are so adept at using denial in our everyday lives that we don't recognize it. Do we see ourselves differently in the mirror than we do in reality? Do we harbor exaggerated notions of our child's academic abilities, our skill on the golf course, or our prowess in accomplishing great trade-in deals at the auto dealership? We may defend these actions as simply slight exaggerations, but aren't they really ways in which we have tried to put a positive spin on life, smoothing the rough edges to bring us a little comfort?

Readers can add their own examples of what might be called "spinning the truth." It may seem harmless in small doses because it protects us from harsh realities: we are getting older and "wider." Our skills aren't what they used to be. Our children may not go to prestigious universities. We aren't as clever with money as we wish.

Oh, yes, we have become so adept at using denial in our everyday lives, we don't think of it as denial. However, it can have a harmful effect even in areas that seem inconsequential. It may keep us from adopting healthy eating habits or maintaining a regular exercise program when we choose not to look closely at our expanding waistlines.

Instead of exaggerating our skills on the golf course or at the auto dealership, it may be time to take a few lessons or ask for advice. And perhaps our child needs extra help in school or even a curriculum adjustment.

Denial and avoidance can protect us when we don't want to face an unpleasant situation, when our busy lives leave no room for additional time, energy, or emotional expenditures. Denial shields us from the fear of Alzheimer's disease.

We are afraid of its uncertain progression. We are afraid of the disruption it will create in our ordered lives. We are afraid we may not be up to the task. We are afraid of losing our loved one. We are afraid it may attack other members of our family, even ourselves. We are also afraid of the stigma still lingering in our society—that there is, somehow, something shameful about a disease that attacks the brain.

ALZHEIMER'S: "THE HIDDEN DISEASE"

Alzheimer's disease is often called "the hidden disease." Individuals with the disease may exhibit no discernible symptoms to the casual observer. They have learned to compensate for their memory loss. Our loved ones are adept at covering up their inability to retrieve the correct words. They laugh when they lose their train of thought. Don't we all have "senior moments"? Their social graces linger even far into the disease, and for many, to the very end. When conversation becomes difficult, they simply listen more and talk less. No wonder it is easy to keep our denial as a comforting barrier from the reality that scares us.

We now share with you some common denial statements and stories. These are true, as are all of the stories in this book. We have heard them over and over while counseling caregivers and their families. The names are changed, the details blended. We betray no one's confidentiality. If you see yourself in one of these stories, you know you are not alone.

THE REFRAIN OF DENIAL RINGS AS A LOUD LAMENT

"Mother is just getting older; there is really nothing wrong with her."

(The deep-down fear) "I can't bear the thought of losing my mother."

"Dad has such a brilliant mind. Everyone has always been in awe of his intelligence."

(Unspoken fear) "I don't want anyone to know his mind is failing. It will make him seem less important. I couldn't bear that."

"My wife looks well and is as beautiful as the day I married her. She's quieter now and clings to me a little more than she used to. I like that."

(A gnawing fear) "If friends know there is something wrong with her mind, will we still be included in the social scene? Does anyone have to know right now? Maybe later, but not now."

Kevin is one of the baby boomers and qualifies as a member of the sandwich generation. He explains his situation: "I have two kids in the turbulent teen years, worries about a promotion, college costs looming. My wife works full-time and heaven knows we need her income. How could we assume the care of her parents? We've got just about all the stress we can handle right now. Is there really anything wrong with my wife's dad? My mother-in-law seems to be taking care of all their needs. We don't want to get involved at this point. Maybe later, but not now."

Debbie is trying to keep an eye on her father. It is not easy. There is a certain sadness in her voice as she relates her concerns: "Dad is getting careless. He's forgetting to throw out food. I'm always cleaning out the fridge. There should be more clothes in the laundry hamper. I don't think he changes clothes every day. I'm afraid he doesn't get enough exercise, and he watches too much TV. When I suggest that he should go to the senior center, he gets upset. My uncle (his brother) thinks he's getting dementia. He claims my dad is always repeating himself and doesn't remember things. I told him Dad is OK; he just misses Mom. She's not there to keep him on the right track. Guess I'll have to watch Dad more closely. I'm sure nothing is really wrong."

When many miles separate the family, distance feeds the denial: "Mom and Dad live at the opposite end of the country from my wife and me. My sister lives near them and she seems to be handling their affairs successfully. Lately she tells me she thinks there is something wrong with Mom. She wants me to come and see for myself. She claims Mom has become argumentative and is sometimes aggressive with Dad. Mom denies that anything is wrong and blames Dad for everything. Dad says she forgets things and Mom says it is Dad who forgets. I talk with Mom every week and she sounds great to me. She tells me everything that is happening. Dad sometimes tells me she mixes things up, but don't we all?! And after all, they are getting older. We can't expect them to act like they did twenty years ago. I have too much going on in my own life to borrow trouble."

The rigid control of the successful businessman or -woman used to getting his or her own way can put a detour on the road to a diagnosis: "Let's wait until something significant develops—no use looking for trouble. Mom looks fine; she's just becoming forgetful, not unusual for a woman of seventy-five. When the time comes, I'll take care of everything. If necessary, Mom can move in with us. My lawyer can handle her affairs. In the meantime we'll keep a good eye on Mom. She'll be OK."

"Our family is scattered all over the country. We all work and have children. No one has enough vacation time or money to deal with Mom's and Dad's daily lives. They say they are doing fine. We want to believe them. We have to believe them!"

"What will I do if my husband can't drive? I haven't been behind the wheel in years. I have forgotten how to drive. We only go to church and the grocery store. Nothing can happen on back roads. We can't lose our independence!"

Some of these family members heeded the advice and council given to them and went on to get a diagnosis. Some family members faced difficulty gaining a family consensus. When a strong family leader remains in denial, it is more difficult for the other members to get professional help for their loved one. If the family can act as a team, it is much easier to deal with troublesome times.

For example, in chapter 2 we tell you what happened when Debbie finally took her dad for an evaluation.

We hear the denial expressed so often at the beginning of the Alzheimer's journey. We remind ourselves that it dogs our footsteps all along the way. We authors have been on this journey. We know it well.

We continue to address each layer of the denial onion and honestly admit there are no absolutes, no perfect solutions to the problems that face us. There are, however, workable choices, positive behaviors, and beneficial attitudes that can create a climate in which living with the disease is made so much easier for both the family and the loved one with AD.

OUT OF DENIAL AND INTO ANGER

On our Alzheimer's journey, it is not uncommon to find ourselves out of denial and into anger. Just as our denial was fed by fear, so is our anger. The fear of the monumental responsibilities that face us may be expressed as anger.

Our anger can develop when we don't get the family support we need. It can simmer when we feel unappreciated. When our favorite recreational activities are curtailed because of caregiving duties, we are upset.

When we don't understand the disease, we expect behaviors that our loved one is now no longer able to give us. We overestimate his abilities and underestimate his cognitive losses. When he fails to understand a simple request, or when he is unable to perform a task today that he could do yesterday, it may provoke our anger. Our loved one's repetitive behavior, his following our every footstep, or "shadowing," may cause frustration that turns to anger when we are suffering from fatigue.

Our own attitude can foster angry feelings within us. We are angry because there is no cure for AD. We feel inadequate for the task of caregiving. "Why me?!" we ask ourselves. And now our anger mingles with guilt.

We feel guilty because we have harbored resentment and anger against our loved one. We feel guilty when we question the quality of care we have given our family member. Is there something we should have done, or could have done better or differently? We probably take ourselves on the biggest guilt trip when we face the prospect of nursing facility placement.

Intellectually we know that guilt is a harmful and destructive emotion. It causes us to dwell in a past we cannot change and even to anticipate a future that may never happen. We need to forgive ourselves for any past mistakes, real or imagined. We did the best we could do at the time.

Just as it is important to recognize our denial all through the Alzheimer's journey, so, too, we must acknowledge our anger and guilt. One of the best places to share our feelings is in a support group. Here we meet companions who are on the same journey. They are not only non-judgmental, but also they understand, for they share our emotional experiences (see chapter 4).

Caring for someone with Alzheimer's disease can cause us to experience inconvenience, stress, annoyance, frustration, and full-blown anger. It is all right to be angry. This is normal and natural. What must concern us is how we express this anger.

Some of us may suppress the anger, another act of denial. We may think we have no anger or that anger is an inappropriate emotion in light of our loved one's disease. So we deny the feelings.

What is anger? Webster defines it as a feeling of extreme displeasure toward someone or something. Don't we feel extreme displeasure toward the disease of Alzheimer's? Of course we do, and it is all right to do so. What is not acceptable is anger directed toward our loved one with AD. For this reason it is our responsibility to learn as much as we can about the disease. We need to understand why our loved one behaves the way he does. We need to learn techniques that will help us deal positively with the challenging behaviors and that will also prevent angry behaviors from our loved one.

When our anger is directed toward family members who seem not to appreciate our caregiving or are reluctant to offer their help, it is time for a reminder: we can only control ourselves.

Exercise is a great stress reliever. When Evelyn experienced extreme frustration, she tried to work it off by completing chores inside and outside of the house. It was not unusual to see Evelyn raking leaves at 9 PM or shoveling sidewalks after dark. Keeping a journal is another way to express anger without hurting anyone. We can find words for our anger, unload our deepest fears, and admit our mistakes.

We need to accept our feelings of anger and guilt as natural. Instead of denying them, we need to understand them. We are angry; we are losing our loved one. We are losing the safe haven of "the usual." The future is uncertain. Can we trust our ability to cope with the difficulties ahead? At times, it is natural to become overwhelmed by a desire to escape our responsibilities. We are not alone! Others have felt this way, too. We need not feel guilty.

As important as it is to take good care of our loved one, it is equally important to take good care of ourselves. As caregivers, we are not being selfish when we put a high priority on our rest, recreation, and laughter. In doing this, we become better at coping successfully with our feelings of anger and guilt. We are more able to develop a positive attitude when dealing with life's vicissitudes. It takes a strong desire and lots of practice to remain in a positive mode while seeking solutions to life's problems. An old New England saying gives us some wise advice: "You cannot control the wind, but you can adjust your sails."

Let us start that adjustment by moving from denial to action. We often remain in denial because we don't know what to do, or we convince ourselves there is nothing we *can* do. We authors would like to dispel that notion as we outline positive actions that will help us get out of the shadow of denial. We must stop holding on to the life that *was* in order to deal with the life that *is*. We must plan for the future.

Positive action, positive attitude—these we owe to the one we love, and to ourselves. In subsequent chapters we will help you, the reader, move from denial to action, which we hope will lead you to acceptance.

Chapter Two

"We Define the Monster"
Alzheimer's Disease

You gain strength . . . and confidence by every experience in which you really stop to look fear in the face. . . . You must do the thing you cannot do.

—Eleanor Roosevelt

John was a meticulous craftsman. When it came time to redecorate, he was the chosen painter. In Evelyn's estimation, no professional could ever match his ability. She was waiting patiently for him to retire because then he planned to paint a bedroom and a bathroom. John explained that once he retired, the job would be easier for him because he would have whole days to work. It was fortunate that Evelyn was patient, because after his retirement she waited and waited and waited. John had one reasonable excuse after another: "I'll start when the days are warmer and the windows can be opened all day." "Are you sure that's the color you want?" "I need to find all my tools." "After I straighten out our investments, I will begin the project."

John never did paint the bedroom or the bathroom. "Straightening out the finances" was the next job that was too difficult for him.

John had always made the travel arrangements. Now it became Evelyn's responsibility. "You do such a good job," John would tell her. He could no longer remember the names of their favorite restaurants. Previously they had taken turns choosing where they would have dinner before the symphony. Now Evelyn chose the restaurant every time. He even let Evelyn order for him—"You know what I like"—because the menu was too confusing.

John was the kind, considerate, loving man he had always been. But gradually, he was letting Evelyn take over the small responsibilities that had been his and letting other jobs, such as painting, go undone.

Evelyn finally faced the fact that something was wrong. She realized that John had not painted because the job was too difficult. There were too many steps in the process: moving furniture, washing walls, mixing paint, and so on.

It took John forever to read a book. He had always been an avid reader; histories and biographies were his favorites. Now when he picked up the book he had started to read yesterday, he had to reread. He didn't remember what he had read yesterday.

In John's own words, "I try so hard." But, no matter how hard he tried, he finally had to admit to Evelyn that she would have to take over the financial responsibilities. He could no longer do even simple math. When she went with him to the tax preparation office and was given instructions by the accountant on how to properly keep the records, she felt overwhelmed. She remembers her thoughts: "I must maintain John's dignity at all costs. I must never let him feel diminished because he has had to relinquish these important duties." What helped more than anything was John's wonderful sense of humor. After the accountant's lessons, John looked at Evelyn and said with a twinkle in his eye, "Well, Honey, from now on you are on your own."

The next day, Evelyn went to John's bank and met with his favorite teller. She and the other tellers were so glad to know that Evelyn was taking over. They had watched John add and re-add his deposit slips, count and recount his checks, spending as much as an hour before walking to the teller's window. They had silently agonized with him. Miss Dell said to Evelyn, "We are so thankful you have relieved him of that dreadful stress."

It was time. Time to find out. Time to give it a name. Evelyn knew and the doctor knew, but the doctor wanted to have a diagnosis from a prominent evaluation center in the area. Yes, John had a disease, and the disease had a name—Alzheimer's.

DEFINING DEMENTIA; DEFINING ALZHEIMER'S

The Alzheimer's Association defines Alzheimer's disease as a progressive brain disorder that gradually destroys a person's memory and ability to learn, reason, make judgments, communicate, and carry out daily activities. (Taken from the "Alzheimer's Disease Fact Sheet—2004.")

Alzheimer's is the most common form of dementia. Dementia is comprised of a group of symptoms that describe a loss of intellectual functioning. The most common dementia symptoms are:

- Memory loss
- Excessive repeating
- Poor judgment
- Difficulty with word retrieval
- Difficulty with abstract thinking

REVERSIBLE CAUSES OF DEMENTIA

There are many causes of dementia. Some causes are reversible if detected and treated early. That should be reason enough to propel a family toward a diagnosis!

Among the many causes of reversible dementia are:

- Vitamin B_{12} deficiency
- Thyroid imbalance
- Prescription drug interactions
- NPH—normal pressure hydrocephalus (fluid in the brain)
- Depression
- Poor nutrition and dehydration
- Alcohol abuse
- Diabetic reactions (sudden drop in blood sugar)
- Electrolyte imbalance
- Kidney failure

These causes of dementia, if diagnosed early, can be successfully treated.

IRREVERSIBLE CAUSES OF DEMENTIA

Some of the irreversible forms of dementia are:

- Alzheimer's disease
- Vascular or multi-infarct dementia, caused by a series of small strokes (infarcts)
- Frontotemporal dementia (Pick's disease)—rare brain disease that resembles AD
- Lewy body disease—exhibits symptoms of both AD and Parkinson's disease
- Parkinson's disease—dementia can occur in the late stages
- Creutzfeld-Jacob disease (CJD)—a rare brain disease caused by infection

As mentioned in the introduction, we will refer to the disease as Alzheimer's disease, or AD. Remember that the other causes of irreversible dementia closely resemble AD. The behaviors of the patients are similar. The tasks of the caregivers are similar.

It is a mistake to think that Alzheimer's disease causes just short-term memory loss. Unfortunately it is far more complicated than that. Although short-term memory loss is one of the most common early symptoms (remember, John could not recall what he read in his book the day before), we should understand "the four As": amnesia, aphasia, agnosia, and aproxia. The four As help us better appreciate what is happening to the brain as the disease progresses, and why certain behaviors are to be expected.

As we stated earlier, this book is not intended to be a clinical, technical examination of the disease, nor will it try to explain in medical terms what is happening in the brain. What is intended is that you, the reader, will better understand the "why" of different, difficult behaviors. You will then be better able to successfully adjust your own behavior when living with, and caring for, your loved one.

THE FOUR As

Amnesia—Short-term memory is lost first. Long-term memory may be lost eventually. Many people with AD enjoy reminiscing far into the disease and enjoy looking at photographs of their youthful days and talking about "home," which often turns out to be their childhood home.

Aphasia—Difficulty with word retrieval is often the first noticeable symptom, then difficulty expressing thoughts and improper use of words follows. Later, the person with AD loses the ability to understand what is being said.

Agnosia—This loss creates behaviors that caregivers often cannot understand. The person with AD is eventually unable to process sensory input. The sensory information may be the ringing of the telephone. The person with AD may be sitting by the phone but will not make any move to answer it. This may cause an impatient response from the family member in the next room who does not understand that her loved one cannot process the sensory input.

The caregiver, who has been using a child's coloring book as an enjoyable afternoon activity for her loved one, may be surprised or upset when one day the person with AD refuses to pick up the crayon. He is not being difficult; he no longer recognizes the familiar object nor knows how to use it. This also explains why he may stop feeding himself or dressing himself, requiring many cues on how to do these common tasks.

Apraxia—This describes the inability to perform coordinated movements, some that we consider automatic: throwing a ball, getting up from a chair or out of bed. The caregiver may have to give step-by-step motion cues to help the person with AD perform a task that was once automatic, but now is very difficult. Unfortunately, the ability to walk may eventually be lost.

It is important to note that these losses happen gradually, in no prescribed fashion, and that the pattern differs from person to person. The particular part of the brain that is involved and the severity of the damage are determining factors in the course of the disease.

Knowledge about these different losses will give the caregiver a better understanding of what is happening to his loved one. He is not trying to be difficult. As John told Evelyn, "I am trying so hard."

Also, behaviors may not be consistent. The family member may be able to perform a certain task today but not tomorrow.

The four As give us an overview of the disease, helping us understand what is happening and what will be happening.

Amnesia, short-term memory loss, usually signals the beginning of the disease. Apraxia, the inability to perform coordinated movements, occurs much later.

THE WARNING SIGNS OF ALZHEIMER'S DISEASE

Let's now look at the initial warning signs that are identified in the Alzheimer's Association's pamphlet "Ten Warning Signs of Alzheimer's Disease."

- Memory loss
- Difficulty performing familiar tasks
- Problems with language
- Disorientation of time and place
- Poor or decreased judgment
- Problems with abstract thinking
- Misplacing things
- Changes in mood or behavior
- Changes in personality
- Loss of initiative

We can see examples of the first two warning signs in John's story. Memory loss was exhibited in his inability to remember passages from the book he was reading. And he did not paint the bedroom because the familiar task had become too difficult.

The following stories, which were shared with Evelyn, illustrate other warning signs:

Sandra gradually lost the use of simple nouns. The fork became the "thing she ate with," the knife was "the thing to cut with," the pen "the thing to write with." Soon all common nouns became "things."

Frank's usually happy demeanor was often replaced by unexplained periods of depression. These uncharacteristic mood swings were unsettling. He began to question all of his actions. When Frank found himself lost one Saturday in the process of doing regular errands, he was frightened. He pulled the car over to the curb in a cold sweat. He truly did not know where he was. After driving slowly for several blocks, he began to recognize familiar landmarks. This harrowing experience, coupled with his disturbing mood swings, sent him to the doctor. He was afraid he was losing his mind. Frank was almost relieved to get the diagnosis of Alzheimer's. He wasn't crazy.

Elaine's mother needed help balancing her checkbook every month. But because of vacations and other interruptions, it had been more than two months since Elaine had helped her mother. It was a bit of a shock to realize that Mother, in this short interval, had sent checks to every nonprofit organization that had sent note paper, cards, and address labels, along with their plea for money. Her mother thought she was obliged to pay for these "gifts." A sizeable portion of her small, monthly income had been given away.

Susan came home one day to find her husband about ready to sign a contract for a security system they could not afford and did not need.

Tom's mother was an independent, capable woman who gave no sign of declining abilities. Tom explained: "I really wasn't looking for problems and had probably ignored small warning signs. But believe me, when I found three months' worth of bills tucked under the cushion of Mother's favorite chair, it was wake-up time for me. It was always a point of honor in our household that all bills were paid on arrival. We never owed a penny to anyone."

Elaine, Susan, and Tom had discovered the poor judgment and the problems with abstract thinking before too much damage was done. Other families have not been as fortunate: Marie gave away or lent large sums of money her family could not recover. Robert signed a contract with a less-than-reliable company for home repairs that he could not afford. Out-of-town family members did not discover the situation until it was necessary to borrow money to pay the contractor.

Evelyn has a humorous story about misplacing things that was told in a somewhat different fashion in Ellen's book, *Between Two Worlds*. Evelyn's mother-in-law had a beautiful two-carat diamond ring that she always put in a safe place. Evelyn was used to being summoned to help find it when Mary could not remember her safe place. It was a little bit like a game: "I wonder where the ring is today?" It had previously been found pinned to her undergarment but also had been hidden in bureau drawers, secret desk drawers, and linen closets. But on the last day that Evelyn agreed to play "find-the-ring," she found it in the refrigerator, pushed into the middle of a stick of butter! Off to the safe deposit box it went.

In all of the experiences just shared, those who showed symptoms of the disease were eventually diagnosed with probable Alzheimer's.

EXAMPLES OF DEMENTIA SYMPTOMS CAUSED BY REVERSIBLE CONDITIONS

Because the warning signs listed above may *not* be symptoms of AD but instead symptoms of a reversible condition, an early diagnosis is extremely important. Reversible disorders are more successfully treated when detected early.

The following stories tell of people experiencing dementia symptoms caused by reversible conditions:

Gloria's mother, Eleanor, was living in a continuing care retirement community in another state. When Eleanor needed minor surgery, Gloria took several days off from work to be with her mother in the hospital. Gloria returned to work only after her mother had safely returned to the healthcare unit in her retirement community. Over the next month Eleanor had several minor flare-ups and was put on various medications to alleviate the adverse symptoms. Gloria admitted to friends that she was a little concerned about her mother's condition. Eleanor had moved from the health center to assisted living. However, Gloria thought Eleanor should be back in her independent apartment by this time. It was quite a shock to Gloria when she received a call from the administrator of the retirement community. He gently advised Gloria of a big change in Eleanor's behavior, which he felt indicated that she should return to the health center rather than independent living. The doctors confirmed this decision. They explained that Eleanor was exhibiting symptoms of dementia. She was very confused, had no immediate memory, and had significant language problems. She could not live independently.

Gloria was disturbed by the number of different medications Eleanor was receiving. She requested family sick leave and again flew back to be by her mother's side. She insisted that the doctors treating her mother review the list of medications and dosages prescribed. After consultation the doctors eliminated one drug, changed another, and revised the dosage of a third. In a week Eleanor's confusion began to clear up. At the end of two weeks, her dementia symptoms were all but gone. By the end of the month, Eleanor was looking forward to moving back to her independent living apartment. It was a learning experience for everyone! A medicine log, including all prescription and over-the-counter drugs with dosage and use, needs to be available for each attending physician to examine. This can prevent a doctor from prescribing adversely interacting drugs.

Eleanor was thankful she had raised a daughter who was an independent thinker with a forceful personality.

We met Debbie and her father, Bill, in chapter 1. Debbie was concerned about her dad's careless hygiene and housekeeping. She could not interest him in activities out of his home. Even Bill's brother was troubled by Bill's memory loss and repetitive behavior. Debbie was able to get her dad to see his doctor. After a thorough physical, which included a detailed history, the diagnosis was depression. Although Debbie realized that her dad missed her mother, she did not connect his behavior to her mother's death. As Debbie explained, "Mother died just over a year ago. Dad handled everything so well. He planned the funeral. It was beautiful. He was our rock—comforting all the family. We were so proud of the way he carried on with the family traditions. He seemed to be adjusting so well. I guess we thought that by this time Dad had passed the grieving stage."

The doctor explained that the grief process does not follow any set pattern. Bill spent his energy comforting others to the point of postponing facing his own grief.

Bill proved to be an extremely cooperative patient. He agreed to attend a grief-counseling group run by a local hospital. He let Debbie plan nutritious meals. He even consented to try medication to give him an initial boost out of his rut of depression.

Bill's brother was the first to comment on the changes in Bill's behavior several months later. "He's much more focused. He is no longer forgetful and repetitive. And I think he is finally doing some honest grieving over his wife's death."

We repeat: Because the warning signs may *not* be symptoms of AD, but instead symptoms of a reversible condition, an early diagnosis is extremely important. Reversible disorders are more successfully treated when detected early.

It is important to note that people with Alzheimer's disease might also suffer from depression. This is quite understandable. As they begin to have difficulty performing basic tasks in addition to experiencing significant memory problems, people with dementia tend to withdraw a bit from the social scene. They may feel a sense of rejection if they can no longer engage in meaningful discussions or participate significantly in family activities. Cognitive problems hamper their ability to share feelings of inadequacy when they realize they can no longer compete, for example, at the bridge table or the Scrabble board. What formerly brought them satisfaction now results in frustration, and even anger.

According to the Alzheimer's Association's fact sheet about depression and Alzheimer's disease, an estimated 20 to 40 percent of those people with AD may experience clinically significant depression. Because a diagnosis may be difficult, it is helpful to have a geriatric physician in charge of our loved one's care from the time of a diagnosis (and even before)—someone who has monitored his behavior over a period of time. The physician may choose to treat the depression with an appropriate drug and/or he may recommend a nondrug treatment. This is treatment that we caregivers should routinely practice whether or not our loved one is diagnosed with depression.

Our loved ones need to be treated with respect at all times. They need to be included in family activities in a way that assures them that they are loved and appreciated. They need to be given as many small choices as possible to give them a feeling of control. They need to be engaged in activities that assure successful outcomes. We must see that they do not get overtired and are not subjected to social gatherings that foster confusion and fatigue. We need always to acknowledge their feelings. They operate best in a structured environment with people who look and act happy. Our loved ones need time outdoors, appropriate exercise, and nutritious meals. We need always to focus on what our loved ones *can* do and tell them they have done well. Tell them they are appreciated; tell them they are loved.

GETTING A DIAGNOSIS

Alzheimer's disease is diagnosed by ruling out all the other causes of dementia. The process could be likened to a thorough physical that no one needs to fear. The following tests are noninvasive.

- A complete medical history
- Patient and (separate) family interview
- Physical exam with complete bloodwork
- Mental status exam
- Neurological exam
- Psychiatric exam
- CAT scan
- MRI

During the separate interviews, John was asked what he had done in the past month. He reported that he had done nothing unusual or out of the ordinary. Meanwhile, Evelyn was describing to her interviewer their marvelous twelve-day trip to France, one that John had thoroughly enjoyed.

Ellen also had a humorous experience with her mother. During the diagnostic process, Ellen's mother was having great difficulty with the questions in the mental status exam. Holding her head high and looking squarely at the doctor, she said, "Young man, when you are my age, you won't know the answers to these questions either!"

These two accounts show us that there can be a lighter side to the diagnostic process.

After Ellen's mother's death, an autopsy indicated that, though she had been diagnosed with AD and Parkinson's, she had actually had Lewy body disease. Her mother was one of the roughly 10 percent who are misdiagnosed. Also, this underscores what we said earlier: other causes of irreversible dementia closely resemble AD.

After all other possible causes of dementia are ruled out, the diagnosis becomes "probable Alzheimer's disease," with an accuracy rate of roughly 90 percent. Today a brain autopsy (postmortem) is the only way to have 100 percent accuracy.

The actual testing procedure may be done by a neurologist or a geriatric specialist, or at a diagnostic center that may be located in any or all of the hospitals in your area. Your family doctor may either make the diagnosis or make a recommendation. Contact your local Alzheimer's office for a list of doctors and centers that specialize in Alzheimer's diagnosis. Choose the doctor or center that you feel suits you and your loved one's particular needs. After the diagnosis you will need to decide who will be the continuing doctor. You may feel comfortable returning to your family doctor. Be sure he or she has geriatric training and experience. If this is not the case, a geriatric specialist may better serve you.

DENIAL STEPS INTO THE PICTURE

With all of this information at hand, it is still possible to be in denial. Let's be honest—no one wants to hear the diagnosis of Alzheimer's disease. We would be far more comfortable believing, "Mom's OK, she just forgets."

It is time to examine some of the reasons denial gives us to avoid facing the truth and reasons for not seeking a diagnosis:

"Why bother having a diagnosis? There is no cure for AD. There is nothing we can do. Let's not upset Dad."

"So Mom forgets a little now and then. Don't we all? No use making a federal case out of it."

"Now, if we could give our aunt some medication to help her, that would be fine. But, I understand the drugs don't help very much. We might as well just continue the way we are. We are really taking good care of Aunt Sue."

"The doctor said Dad was just getting a little senile. It happens to all people as they get older. He told us we needed to be patient with his forgetfulness and watch him a little closer than before."

"Mom won't go to see the doctor. I know she won't. And Mom always gets her own way."

Perhaps you, the reader, have heard one of those denial excuses from a family member. Or perhaps you have had similar feelings. "Mom's too old. It would only upset her. Why worry over a little memory loss? There is nothing we can do."

If you feel this way, you are not alone. Evelyn has heard these arguments stated in a variety of ways over the past twelve years while answering Helpline calls at her local Alzheimer's chapter. Ellen heard similar reasoning when dealing with families in her role as a hospital social worker.

Denial is a common defensive reaction to an unwanted event. Denial protects the body from actual physical harm, but when kept too long, it becomes destructive.

ANSWERING THE DENIAL ARGUMENTS

We need that early diagnosis for several reasons. We need to find out whether the dementia is reversible or irreversible. Remember that reversible dementia, when diagnosed early, can usually be treated successfully. If the diagnosis is Alzheimer's or a related disorder, there are important matters that will need attention.

When Jim, a seventy-two-year-old retired engineer, received his diagnosis of Alzheimer's disease, he told his wife he was not happy about the diagnosis, but he couldn't say that he was surprised. He was aware of the telling symptoms he was experiencing. He knew that now it was time to plan, and the first thing he wanted to do was take that trip to Italy, to see the churches of Rome, the art in Florence, and the opera in Milan. He and his wife had talked about this trip for years. They always said, "When the children are grown and we have retired, we will live it up and take that trip to Italy." Jim decided they could not wait. "We must go now."

Jim confessed he enjoyed his grandchildren more than ever. "This is the first day of the rest of my life," Jim said, reciting a well-worn phrase. "I may not remember it tomorrow, but I sure will *live* today."

Not everyone is able to greet adversity with such aplomb. But there can be no doubt that the positive assurance with which Jim faced his difficult situation helped him, as well as all of his family, as they traveled the bumpy Alzheimer's road. He set the tone. He put as positive a spin as was humanly possible on the situation. He was able to give his family this valuable support because he had an early diagnosis and was still able to understand the situation they all faced.

Another reason for early diagnosis is to be sure all legal, health, and financial decisions are made while the family member with AD is deemed competent. He needs to designate his health agent as durable medical power of attorney. This must be someone he trusts to make decisions pertaining to his health when he is no longer able. Also, he needs to appoint a trusted family member or friend to be given durable financial power of attorney to handle his monetary affairs when he needs this assistance (see appendix).

Many family members stall when faced with this vital step, declaring, "Mother [or Dad] will never give up control of financial or health decisions."

If your loved one is aware of the diagnosis and understands that he has a progressive disease, it may be easier to convince him of the importance of putting his affairs in order while he is able. It also helps if he is not the only one seeking these documents. Actually, all adults should consider having in place healthcare decisions, which include a designated healthcare agent, healthcare instructions, and a living will. In some states they are called advance directives, and the proper forms can be obtained from the office of the state attorney general. Your local Alzheimer's Association office as well as local hospitals may have copies of the documents. You may choose to have several family members fill out these forms with your loved one. It can be a cooperative effort so he does not feel singled out.

In the same manner, completing the durable power of attorney documents may be a joint effort with Mom or Dad and one or two siblings together in the lawyer's office. Wills can be updated at the same time. It is important to choose an eldercare lawyer who understands current laws and knows what legal steps need to be taken to protect the family. The lawyer can assure your family member that he is making the proper decision in obtaining the durable general power of attorney documents. The lawyer is the professional advising his adult client. This is far different from an adult child telling his or her parent what to do.

If your loved one has an early diagnosis, her doctor may choose to start her on one of these FDA-approved drugs: donepezil (Aricept), rivastigmine (Exelon), or galantamine (Razadyne). These drugs do not cure or stop the progression of Alzheimer's. Some patients taking these drugs may experience temporary improvement. The drugs may cause them to feel and act brighter, and they may slow the progression of the disease. For optimum effect, these drugs need to be taken in the early stages of AD. The drugs, while safe, may cause side effects. Many patients experience no discernable improvement while taking them.

With an early diagnosis, patient and doctor can develop a meaningful relationship. The doctor will have a baseline with which to compare future behaviors. Families should look for board certified doctors with training in geriatric medicine. A list of such doctors can be obtained from local hospitals. As stated earlier, the diagnostic center may suggest a competent geriatric doctor, with an office close to the family's home, to be the continuing doctor. The patient needs to be seen on a regular basis. It is important to note that while the drugs that can be prescribed for early-stage AD may not be effective in every case, there are medications that can be used to alleviate some of the other disturbing symptoms of AD, such as depression and agitation. Sometimes irregular sleep patterns can be corrected.

Good geriatric physicians will not tell you, "Your mother's getting a little senile. It happens to all of us when we get older." They do not use the term *senility*. They know that AD is not just a part of aging. It is a disease.

Consider this. A friend (and reader of this book in its early stages) is a ninety-five-year-old nun. She is a former high school principal and teacher of English. Sister is "sharp as a tack," has a marvelous sense of humor, keeps abreast of all current events, and walks straight and strong, hardly needing the cane she sometimes uses, just in case. Lydia is one hundred years old, but looks about seventy-five. She resides in a lovely retirement community where she participates regularly in Bible study classes. When she comes to the large meeting hall, she parks her walker in the far corner of the room and walks with ease to a seat near the speaker. Sister and Lydia would not like to think that because of their age they would be described as "a little senile." Remember, it is not "old-timers' disease." It is Alzheimer's disease, named after the doctor who discovered it, Alois Alzheimer.

On the other hand, it is true that the greatest risk factor for AD is age. About 10 percent of those sixty-five and older are at risk of developing the disease. This risk factor increases to about 50 percent at age eighty-five. These statistics tell us that not everyone who grows older gets AD.

One of the more comfortable denial statements is the one about "the stubborn mother who won't go to the doctor." Why is this such a "comfortable" statement? The daughter explains, "It's not my fault that Mother isn't being diagnosed. My stubborn mother is to blame." In fact, the problem may not be the stubborn mother but the adult child in comfortable denial, who won't face the difficult situation squarely. We would like to offer an approach that has worked for others. Evelyn calls it "rearranging reality." (See chapter 6.)

Mother balks at the idea of visiting the doctor. Daughter talks with the doctor and/or the nurse, explains the problem she is having, and asks them to help her with her plans. Daughter explains to Mother that she herself needs to go to the doctor but doesn't want to go alone. "Mother, would you please go with me? It would make me feel much more comfortable." Daughter can invent some vague symptoms (not serious, but perhaps worrisome) if necessary. At the doctor's office, Mother and Daughter go into the examining room together. The nurse takes Daughter's vital signs, then suggests this is a good time to include Mother. Daughter needs blood work—might as well include Mother. Then the doctor can talk with Mother and explain why he/she wants to follow up with more tests. As in the case of the lawyer, a professional is advising a client; here the physician is advising the patient. Daughter is not telling Mother what to do. This scenario does depend on a supportive physician, but this basic plan has worked.

Another approach is to examine the reasons behind Mother's reluctance to visit the doctor. She may always have been a determined woman, dictating her own rules. But in this instance is it really her stubborn nature that is causing her behavior? Indeed, it is very likely that it is Mother's own denial, fed by fear, which keeps her from the doctor. She may be stubborn. She is also afraid. The family needs to choose carefully the person to approach Mother. That person should be reassuring but also firm. Mother knows whom she can dominate. Give her choices: which doctor, what day, who will accompany her, what will she wear. Look for ways to alleviate her fear and gain her confidence. Always give her some control and maintain her dignity.

TO TELL OR NOT TO TELL?

Today it is hard to believe that any adult has not heard of Alzheimer's disease. Families openly share the diagnosis. Many of us have friends, family, or neighbors with the disease. We read newspapers and magazine articles about the ongoing research and clinical trials searching for a vaccine, cure, or advanced treatment. Authors are using the disease in story plots we read in novels or see on TV.

Fortunately Alzheimer's has gradually come out of the closet. We openly discuss the disease and plan for the future. We work for a cure as we participate in local Alzheimer's fund-raisers, such as walks, galas, and golf tournaments. The disease becomes less frightening and more manageable. We look at it squarely. It is not a disgrace to have a disease of the brain. It doesn't mean we are crazy. There are positive steps we can take after the diagnosis and through the course of the disease.

Families are still asking, "Should we tell Mom that the diagnosis is Alzheimer's disease?" Many doctors feel that all of their patients should be told. If it is early in the disease, this gives them the opportunity to participate in the legal, financial, and health plans. Like Jim, patients may decide to live life a little differently, savoring each day. Remember Frank? He was relieved to know that he had a disease with a name. He wasn't crazy. There are others like Frank who need to clarify all the uncertainty.

Some doctors leave the decision to tell or not to tell up to the family. Many patients are not surprised when they learn of the diagnosis. They know something has been wrong for quite a while, more than those joked-about "senior moments." They may not like the diagnosis, but it fits their symptoms. It may be easier to reason with these patients when it comes time for daycare or giving up driving.

When Mother, Dad, husband, or wife initially refuses to go to the doctor, the reason is probably denial. They know something is wrong, but they choose to make all the necessary excuses to cover their mistakes. Eventually they convince themselves that nothing is really wrong. If the diagnosis is shared with them, it should be done with great care. The loving spouse may be able to take the fear from the situation as he tells his wife, "We will face this disease together. I will always love you. We still have good years ahead." The loving daughter will want to remind Mother or Dad that the family will give its support and love. But more than that, the family members need to be assured that life can still be meaningful and productive.

Ann tells how she helped her mother and herself after the diagnosis. "We all knew there was something wrong with Mom. My sister Florence and I almost hated to find out for sure, but we knew that if Mom had Alzheimer's we had to plan for the future. After we found out, you know what really struck me? It was my belief that we had to let Mom know right away how important she was to us, how much we loved her. Mom had tried so hard to hide her memory loss, as if it were something to be ashamed of. We told her she had AD. We let her know it didn't matter. She was still Mom and we loved her just as she was. Florence and I made sure we told her all the important events in our lives. We asked her advice, told her jokes, took her to see funny movies, and took her shopping to help us pick out clothes. It wasn't that we were doing things differently, but the things we did took on greater importance."

If your family member is not in the early stage of the disease, she may not understand the diagnosis and may not remember it after she is told. You may feel that knowing the diagnosis will cause anger directed at the family or cause such an upset as to make the telling unwise. It is the family's decision. In most cases sharing this diagnosis is probably the best course to take. What is most important is the way in which it is done.

We hope we have dispelled the notion that there is "no reason to get a diagnosis, for there is nothing we can do anyway." We have provided sound evidence of the critical importance of early diagnosis.

It is time to put financial and legal affairs in order. It is time to secure a competent geriatrician. It is time to become educated about the disease. It is time to gather the family together to plan for the journey ahead. We authors have walked the walk, each more than once. We will be offering you our best advice and companionship along the way.

Chapter Three

"Mom's OK, She Just Forgets"
Denial and the Family Unit

Love is not love which alters when it alteration finds.

—William Shakespeare

THE "FAMILY" AND DEMENTIA

In this chapter, we will be talking about Alzheimer's disease, denial, and the family. Families come in many shapes, forms, and configurations. Whatever constitutes "family" to the reader, is family. The ability of denial to burrow into a family system will be discussed in the different scenarios that are presented in this chapter. We cannot cover every possible family situation, but we trust that readers will be able to fill in the blanks and will be able to see themselves in some of the scenarios.

For most of us, most of the time, family is a word that has a warm, positive connotation. Webster calls family, "a group of people related by ancestry or marriage; relatives." That definition reminds us that all those related by marriage, both the in-laws and the "outlaws" are included. Some who are considered family members are related only by love. Groupings can be unique.

Family members can bring one another joy and feelings of security. Conversely, toxic relationships can bring anguish. A lesson we each learn at some time in our life is that family relationships can both bless and burn. We hope, in this chapter, to help families realize that there are blessings even in the midst of pain.

When Alzheimer's disease sneaks into the picture, the very closest and loving of families may threaten to come apart at the seams. The temptation is to go into an emotional fetal position. Tempting though that may be, your guides throughout this book, Ellen and Evelyn, are not going to let that happen. All of us will continue to stare Alzheimer's down. *We will not allow our hearts to be contaminated by fear.* For it is fear that is the parent of denial, and our mission is to conquer denial.

Some form of dementing illness has entered the life of our loved one and is also affecting our lives. We may not, as yet, have definite information, but we know something is wrong. It is a devastating feeling. We must try to remember that countless people have trod these labyrinthine ways before us. We are not alone.

The task at hand is to bring the family together, first to arrange for an accurate diagnosis, then to begin planning for appropriate care. This chapter will lay out workable approaches for families who find themselves in many dilemmas, including the prevalent "communication crisis." Families who work well together will have an easier time, perhaps, but dysfunctional families may actually gain more from this whole experience. Adversity has the power to bring about growth.

Families are, by nature, made up of different personality types. We all know families who have "the helpless one," "the know-it-all," "the busy one" (his or her work and time are more important than ours). Then there are the eldest, middle, or youngest child syndromes. These personalities can really be a nuisance or just blips on the screen. Our advice: make every effort to keep them at the "blip level."

In planning for a loved one, before the diagnosis or at any stage of the Alzheimer's journey, everyone's voice should be heard to the greatest extent possible. Each member of the family is responsible for, and entitled to, input. We must make sure everyone is not just *listening* but is also *hearing* what is being said. That means listening to one person at a time without interrupting. It means digesting what has been said and then responding. Although each family member's needs must be considered, there are times when individual needs must be put on the back burner. It's not always easy; it is really a balancing act.

Each family member should be respected as an individual, and everyone must try to avoid scapegoating anyone in order to funnel off some anger. (We can be the generators or receivers of this kind of behavior long before we realize what is happening.) Listening to one another respectfully and considering everyone's opinion is critical. Also, everyone should contribute to the research necessary to solve the particular problem at hand. Without information, fear is fed. Lack of knowledge can also spawn anger and frustration.

We can all have hope that our families can feel comfortable as a group and also as individuals. If each member can manage to keep a sense of humor and a positive attitude, dealing effectively with one another cannot only be achieved but also can be very rewarding.

As the name of this book implies, we present the following scenario: (Obviously, it can be Mom or Dad who is "OK and just forgets.")

SCENARIO ONE: A SUCCESS STORY

The family gathers to talk about Mom. She is a widow and has been managing very well on her own for more than fifteen years. Her daughter lives nearby but is at work all day. Concerned neighbors have reported to the daughter that her mother has been seen wandering the neighborhood, seeming lost or in a fog. A friend has reported that Mom has come home from the store a couple of times recently without her groceries, leaving them in the basket near the door of the grocery store.

The out-of-state son's first reaction is, "We all do that kind of stuff. Mom's OK, she just forgets."

Is that the case, or is this a wake-up call?

The daughter is concerned. She has noticed that Mom is forgetting a lot of things. Appointments are missed, lunches with friends are forgotten. Most alarming is that Mom no longer seems to care about her appearance. She wears the same outfit every day and she used to be so particular about what she wore. It seems that this involves more than simple forgetting.

After much discussion and citing specific examples to her brother, the daughter convinces him that something must be done. Mom's evaluation by a geriatric psychiatrist results in a diagnosis of "dementia of the Alzheimer's type." The two siblings each have young children and they feel that Mom would probably not do well living in either of their homes. It would be too noisy. Mom likes quiet and now she needs quiet. They decide to look into an assisted living facility after making plans to have someone stay with Mom while they are exploring.

Other family members, friends, and neighbors pitch in and offer assistance until placement can come about. Mom does not resist and seems almost relieved to know there is a diagnosis. She had been feeling confused and overwhelmed all of the time.

Calling this a "success story" may sound a bit exaggerated, but it truly is an example of one. Whenever agreement can be reached within a family without too much time and trouble, it is good. Enlisting the assistance of friends and neighbors is good, too. They can be of paramount importance in helping to make things run smoothly. They can stay with our confused loved one, run an errand, or just be there for support. Families who have willing and helpful friends and neighbors are very fortunate.

"But wait a minute," we hear, "we can't just 'put Mom away' or 'place her in a nursing center'—whatever euphemisms you want to use! She won't go and we can't force her."

This is a perfectly understandable reaction. Making a transition as smoothly as the one discussed above is rare. The good news is that it does happen. However, if it is too soon for a nursing center, we can enhance our loved one's life by exploring the possibility of a daycare program. (See chapter 8.) Or, we can even back up one step, if necessary, and have a home-care companion in the home for a few weeks before trying daycare. This way, the changes will happen gradually. It is true, though, that some people with dementia are happy to be in a facility that is geared to their specific needs. If it is the right facility, it can be accepted more easily by both family and loved one. (See chapter 10.)

SCENARIO TWO: A UNIVERSAL STORY

Nearly everyone dealing with a loved one with dementia can relate to this story. There are always the nonbelievers—friends or other family members who don't see anything wrong with our confused loved one, even when the disease is quite advanced. More of the "Mom's OK" phenomenon! One daughter, Jean, told the story of her siblings who continued to doubt that their mother had dementia.

*Their denial is understandable, because news of this sort is a devastating blow
and not easy to accept.*

*Jean's siblings lived out of state and Mom often visited, making the trip
alone. Enough time had passed since the last visit for Mom to have become
noticeably more confused. Jean decided to send Mom by bus on her next visit.
The family met Mom at the bus station and thought she seemed OK. It was
amazing how well she could hold it together for a short visit. Even after two days
the family was still puzzled. (Denial had moved in and was trying to take up
permanent residence!) Jean called and asked if they would mind having Mom
stay a little longer. The family agreed. The next night, when everyone else was
in bed, Mom escaped and walked onto a nearby highway. Unharmed, she was
found by the police, not only wandering, but actually hitchhiking!*

*Finally the rest of the family had to admit that Mom was doing all the things
Jean had been telling them about. Jean felt vindicated.*

In this scenario, Mom was a woman in her late sixties with very strong
social graces. Having her daughter put her on the bus for her family to meet
her at the other end was something she could still manage. The "social
grace" phenomenon is discussed throughout this book. It can cause a situation with a loved one to seem bizarre, almost a "now you see it—now you
don't" phenomenon!

Jean had the right idea to arrange for the doubting family member (or
members) to spend as much time as possible with Mom. Time has a way of
taking care of these things. The truth unfolds!

We authors want to suggest as many ways as possible to solve problems
and gently nudge each family member a little further on the path from
denial to acceptance. Readers who are seeking solutions may be the only
ones in their families to recognize that something is wrong with a loved
one. On the other hand, the whole family may already be aware that there
is a diagnosis of dementia. Either way, there will probably be a few bumps
along the way.

As we move forward in this chapter on denial and the family unit, we
are on a journey together. We will try to put denial a little further behind
us, or put it in its proper place, as we become more conscious of acceptance—which is our goal. But how do we overcome denial? Can it ever be
overcome? We know denial is related to fear; the only thing that overcomes

fear is to bring to light that which is causing it. Bring it out in the open; don't run from it. Gather information. The more we learn, the more we can process, the more we will adapt to the situation. If nothing more, we will grow accustomed to dealing with dementia and it will lose some of its power.

SCENARIO THREE: EARLY-ONSET AD

A woman in her fifties is experiencing a notable personality change. Tragically, it is a case of early-onset Alzheimer's disease. (Only 5 to 8 percent of all Alzheimer's cases are early onset.) Distinguishing the terms early-stage *and* early-onset *is important. Early-onset AD means the disease is diagnosed in someone under age sixty-five. Early-stage indicates that someone with AD is in the beginning stage of the disease. The term* late-onset *refers to people who display symptoms after sixty-five, and* late-stage *is when a person is in the later stages of AD. (Research has shown early-onset Alzheimer's to have a greater genetic component than late onset.) The woman's husband and children are devastated. They are not a particularly close-knit family, but they are not hostile. They agree to meet. Trying to discuss the situation rationally, they are overcome by emotion and spend most of the time trying to comfort one another. Mom has no insight as to what is happening to her. She has lost much of her self-awareness and thinks she is fine. Her family wants to believe that she is really OK and that the diagnosis is wrong. They try hard to help her with reminders and cueing, but they cannot save Mom from the labyrinth. Added to their denial is guilt that is so often fed by feelings of helplessness. The out-of-town siblings say, "It's impossible; Mom is too young for this to happen!" Finally, their attitude becomes, "There's nothing that can be done for Mom's problem, so why not just leave things alone and ignore it as much as possible."*

Fortunately, in this scenario, Mom has a sister with a background in nursing. The sister is determined to help the family get through the denial. Feeling as if she is doing something worthwhile helps her keep her own fear in check. Finally she convinces the family that their attitude is not productive. She explains that AD research is advancing rapidly; there are medications available that may stabilize their mother in the early stages of the disease, at least for a period of months and possibly longer. Medication has been known to help for up to two years. It is always possible that a breakthrough toward a cure could occur during that time. Once an ability is lost, it cannot be recovered. With no intervention, the descent is insidious and definite. The sister's efforts to convince the family to take Mom in for a complete medical workup are finally successful. Everyone feels better, even in the midst of this adversity, because they are, at least, "doing something." And from there, some real planning can begin.

Here we see a family that is not particularly close, one that is tightening up at a difficult time. We hope that fragmented families will be reintegrated at the time when such a crisis strikes. This can, and does, happen. Families not only "go" through the process of dealing with a loved one with Alzheimer's, but also they "grow" through the process. Growth and healing can often evolve out of pain. Family units that have been close will usually (but not always) have a smoother experience when coming together to plan for the loved one. Over time, they have developed the skills necessary to communicate effectively and to organize an approach to the problem. This model is more the exception than the rule, but even previously dysfunctional families can and do pull together when the going gets tough.

SCENARIO FOUR: MOM AND DAD IN DENIAL

Mom has been in denial. Dad has been in denial. Dad now has a diagnosis of AD-type dementia. He is retired and has recently become an unsafe driver. There have been two accidents and he has lost his way several times. Mom has her own health issues and is not able to assume all the extra responsibility. One daughter lives nearby. Other children live out of town. Some of the children are more informed than others about what is happening. Being aware intellectually does not always translate into emotional understanding and acceptance of the situation. The children, though middle-aged adults, are reluctant to confront Mom with the fact that she can no longer manage Dad's care.

Here is an attempt at a recipe for success. After the initial shock that Mom is no longer able to care for Dad, the family members (including spouses) should make every effort to arrange their schedules to come together as a unit. Clearing work calendars, taking family leave, making travel plans—whatever it takes—must be done to convene that much-needed family powwow. Relatives may be scattered all over the country and even all over the world. Or there may be only one or two who make up the whole family and who live practically next door.

Be sure to have someone take notes—or better yet, tape the entire meeting. Then there can be no selective memories of what was said.

The family finally comes together after making arrangements for Mom to be involved in an activity with Dad and a friend. This way Mom will be otherwise occupied and not be obsessing about what is going on at the family meeting. She can join in later. It would be unfair to include Mom until the family has reached some agreement and can present cogent suggestions about such things as daycare, assisted living, or nursing home placement—whatever best meets both Mom's and Dad's needs. Once Mom is included, brought up to speed, and has had her say, Dad should also be included. Out of respect, no matter how impaired Dad is, it is important for everyone to lovingly explain to him what the consensus is in terms of planning for him.

Three daughters, two with spouses, and one son and his wife, sit down to share information, discuss, and plan. One of the daughters lives ten minutes from Mom and Dad. The other children live out of state. Margo, Janet, and Don feel that they must acknowledge the deeper involvement of Carol, who lives nearby. Immediately there is tension.

Here, the siblings who live out of town thought they were dealing with the primary caregiving sibling. "You live here, Carol, and are more involved than we are. So we'll let you start off with your thoughts and ideas." Unfortunately this is interpreted by Carol as, "We're letting you have more to say in exchange for more involvement, for doing more for Mom and Dad." While essentially true, the one mistake Carol makes is to assume this means the other three will not be helping at all. Because nerves are on edge and tempers are a little short from the tension, voices rise and an argument begins.

Carol says angrily, "You guys are real jerks if you think I'm going to continue being the workhorse here!"

What is really being said? Carol has felt overwhelmed with all the extra responsibility for quite some time and has reached the breaking point. Even though she doesn't live with Mom and Dad, she has been doing a lot for them. She works and has a busy life of her own. She is the classic tired, harried caregiver.

This outburst shocks everyone into the realization that they had better try to keep their cool and move on with their discussion. They realize they must make a greater effort to take a hard look at the situation and do some real planning. "OK," says Don. "It'll be easier if one of us acts as coordinator to *get things going. I'll do it because I'm the eldest and Carol is clearly tired at this point."*

They all agree.

It is important to insert here that each situation will be different, in terms of selection of the main spokesperson/leader. Sometimes it is automatically the elder sibling who may have always had good family leadership skills; sometimes it is the person most involved with the day-to-day care; sometimes it is the sibling closest, either logistically or emotionally, to Mom and/or Dad. It may even turn out that a beloved daughter-in-law or son-in-law with good managerial skills can be more objective. (We authors recommend whatever works for each family—and only the "collective you" can figure that out. The most important thing is to take the necessary time to think things through and discuss everything thoroughly. Giving all of this your precious time is crucial to success!)

With Don in charge, the group starts to make progress.

Carol expresses her fear of being left holding the bag. Her outburst earlier is a strong indicator of physical and emotional exhaustion. She reminds everyone that she loves Mom and Dad but that she also has a busy life to lead. She makes the clear statement, "There is only so much any one human being can do."

Hours later the meeting finally ends. Some concrete things are accomplished, and plans are made. In a nutshell, the out-of-state siblings agree to pitch in a certain amount of money each month to obtain homemaker services, hoping that Mom will allow someone in the home. This will cut Carol's duties in half. One of the siblings agrees to pitch in by spending a weekend a month with Mom and Dad. Don plans to keep track of all of the finances by computer. That will also be a big help.

Coming to agreement about allocating tasks to different people should be done as quickly as possible. This is where denial can raise its head once more. If it all takes too much time, the family's ability to organize and proceed with a plan of care in the most effective and efficient way is undermined. As a family, the members must try to remember that they are adults who care about one another. They must be ready to assume tasks. The family in this scenario did a good job.

Again, after the rough plan has been outlined among the adult children as to who will do what, Mom can be included. This will prevent her from having any feelings of either being ignored or being under attack at the family meeting. There may be some families who wish to include Mom in the whole process. This is fine, as long as the decision is mutually agreed upon. Otherwise, the whole atmosphere of the meeting will be negatively affected.

Other ideas for allocating tasks for family members include driving, accompanying Mom and Dad to appointments, doing household chores, food shopping, and so on. These things get done when children live nearby. But friends and neighbors can also help. And we've shown that family members can contribute even when they live out of state. They can do research via the Internet and can even keep track of or manage finances long distance. Computers make a lot of things possible. E-mail is a great way to keep all family members up to date on what is happening. Teleconferencing is also a great idea.

We can't say this too often: being as organized as possible and working together as efficiently as possible toward a plan of care is the way to ease the tension and pain.

In this scenario, it is obvious that the natural tendency is to focus completely on Dad. In the beginning Dad is the one who needs the most attention. Then comes Mom. And then comes Carol. Remember the mantra, *I can't take care of you unless I take care of myself.* Everyone's needs should be considered. It is the only way to prevent emotional burnout for all family members when dealing with a situation as difficult as Alzheimer's disease.

Rather than exploring every possible task and family configuration, suffice it to say that now we have seen clearly that coming together is critically important. This is the real opportunity for a family to try to move through the stages of denial as a unit. There will rarely be two families that will have the same reaction to the situation, but at least everyone can be on the same page in terms of the facts. And again, everyone can and should have input into the planning. (This is also a good hedge against having denial take up residence!)

If this scenario had involved a widowed parent with dementia, arrangements should have been made to have a trusted friend or professional aide stay with her while the family met. Thus all can be free to speak openly without being afraid of causing more confusion for the parent.

The outcomes of all of the scenarios in this chapter have many possible variables, and each may open up another can of worms. For example, if the wife/mother refuses to "allow a stranger into her house to help," there goes the cleaning person or homemaker plan. Sometimes even the idea of letting a helpful neighbor get involved to do a chore goes out the window. Mom may feel she can't reciprocate, so she refuses the offer of help. If the offer is presented at a later time, she may accept it.

Nevertheless even a rough plan is better than no plan. Naturally there will be successes and failures along the way.

More space has been given to the above scenario because it is the most prevalent. Sometimes it is Mom who has dementia and sometimes it is Dad. Unfortunately there are times when dementia strikes both in similar time frames, bringing double trouble (and double the denial) and necessitating a double portion of the tips offered here.

Guardianship is another important issue to touch on in this chapter. Our four scenarios involve family members and close friends. If there is not a family member or friend willing to take responsibility for the person with dementia, and the person becomes so impaired that he or she can no longer function, a real problem arises. It may then become necessary to have the person adjudicated incompetent by a court of law and have a guardian appointed through the department of social services. Guardianship can involve one or two people as guardian(s) of person and guardian(s) of property. One person may serve as both or there may be two appointees.

Readers deserve kudos for reading this far, for having the determination to follow through with something as unpleasant as dealing with a loved one's dementia. The natural tendency is to run away from the whole scene. It is perfectly legitimate to struggle, sometimes desperately, with the countless feelings and anxieties that arise. We who have been there have done lots of struggling, too. Ellen fought accepting the diagnosis of Alzheimer's for her mother and aunt for a long time, always hoping for another diagnosis or cause. "Perhaps it's from the high blood pressure, perhaps it's ministrokes. How about a vitamin deficiency or depression? There must be something the doctors have missed!" We are all terrified of the diagnosis because of what it might mean for our loved one *and* for us. "Will people start watching us to see if we are showing signs of memory loss?"

When we finally confront our own fears, we realize that it is the welfare of our loved one that matters, not what label the disease is given. Ellen, having the advantage of being a social worker in a hospital setting and dealing with dementia daily in her case load, was able to calm herself and establish a plan for treatment. When she reached that stage, she knew she had taken some of the wind out of the denial. She had given denial a resounding kick out the door!

THE IMPORTANCE OF PLANNING

At this point, we can all afford to stop, take another look at the situation, and try to adjust attitude and perspective. When planning as a family for our loved one, we must try to draw on the attitudes of the more positive people in the group. Again, it is so important to try to keep our sense of humor—not an easy assignment when in the midst of the crisis. Once again, all we can do is try.

The most important thing is to move on with the planning. When it comes to dividing up the tasks, if neighbors and friends are involved in the care of our loved one, so much the better. It is imperative to garner all possible assistance. Shopping, running errands, taking Mom or Dad to a medical appointment or out for a walk or drive—are all helpful interventions. Making a trip to the library or bookstore to collect as much information as possible would be helpful. Contacting the Alzheimer's Association should be a priority. There are many ways in which these dedicated, experienced, caring people can offer advice and solace. They've been there before and have done whatever we are in the midst of doing. (See the appendix for the main number of the Alzheimer's Association. They will connect you to the chapter nearest you.)

As we said in chapter 2, we should be planning for the inevitable. We are living in times when preplanning for catastrophic events can save a great deal of stress and anguish. There is no downside to having advance directives (living wills) and to having a loved one appointed as durable medical power of attorney, as well as durable power of attorney for finances.

Everyone should be doing it, whether or not Alzheimer's is involved. A very effective way to navigate this situation is to have Mom and Dad both complete their directives and wills, thereby preventing the loved one with Alzheimer's from feeling like the "identified patient." Or when it is the adult child accompanying the parent to the attorney's office, the child can file his/her own papers along with Dad or Mom, again to prevent anyone from feeling singled out. It works! (Just make sure that the appointed durable powers of attorney, both financial and medical, include someone other than Mom and Dad.)

As difficult as it may seem, in a situation filled with potential difficulties, families should keep their eyes open for some hidden blessings or silver linings along the way. One such blessing may be that the loved one never has to know about a serious illness suffered by another family member, or even the death of a loved one. As sad and heartrending as dementia is, it can serve as a cloak of protection from anxiety for those affected, especially if they have been worriers. This happened with Ellen's mother. She became content when the dementia reached a certain point. It is the family that suffers because of "the long good-bye" and the feelings of loss. In cases where the confused loved one seems fairly peaceful, the families can take heart in knowing that their loved one is not suffering.

We may say, philosophically, that the cup of life is filled only to the halfway mark. It is up to us to decide whether the cup is half-full or half-empty. We cry when we are sad, but we cry also when we are happy. Sometimes we laugh so hard we cry. There are tears involved at both ends of the spectrum of human emotion.

"Love is not love which alters when it alteration finds." Shakespeare knew how to cut through to the central truths of life. Love that is real doesn't change when the person changes, especially when that change is beyond anyone's control. True love has many faces. The emotional and the romantic face must give way to the more durable face of "love in action"— doing for our loved one. This is the highest form of love.

It has been said that the way we find happiness in life is not by what we *get* but by whom we *become*. As caregivers, we embark on "the hero's journey." A good antidote to the fear and pain sometimes experienced on this journey is gratitude. We can try to see the cup as half-full by concentrating more on what is left than what is lost. Our loved one is still the same person, though now cloaked in a personality-altering illness. Important concepts to take away from this chapter, and every chapter in this book, are the sacredness, dignity, and uniqueness of each human being.

Alzheimer's causes a person's brain to be slowly destroyed, analogous to the damage caused to the body due to lack of insulin in diabetes. Fortunately for diabetics, insulin replacement can make their lives nearly normal. It is our hope that an equally effective intervention will soon be found for Alzheimer's disease, even if that intervention involves nothing more than holding the disease back for as long as possible.

One last caveat. There may be one or more family members who will never move far enough out of denial to become a part of "the team." We must accept this and not fight it. We must not let it cause us to become angry. We must not allow this family member to hamper our progress. Someday he or she may willingly join our team. Leave the door open and the welcome mat out.

For the family darkened by Alzheimer's disease, sometimes the truth dawns slowly that some clouds are not replaced by silver linings. Not every journey is a smooth one, but thankfully, most journeys can be improved with knowledge. In reality, denial among family members can raise its head throughout the course of the illness, as new decisions about care of the loved one need to be made. But nevertheless, family members can be a wonderful source of support for one other. If nothing more, they may eventually all pitch in together to give denial a permanent boot out the door.

Chapter Four

"I Can't Take Care of You unless I Take Care of Myself" Caring for the Caregiver—Part 1

Beyond a wholesome discipline, be gentle with yourself.

—Max Ehrmann

The job of caregiving is too difficult to do alone. No matter how capable we are, no matter how independent we are, we cannot, we must not, try to walk this road alone. We cannot be effective caregivers unless we take care of ourselves. Unless diffused, the stress of caregiving can lead to significant health problems. If the primary caregiver becomes ill, what then?

There are many pieces to our support network and all are important. We need to have them all in place. At various stages on the Alzheimer's journey, one may be more important than another.

GETTING PROFESSIONAL HELP

After the initial diagnosis, we need to build a support system starting with a trusted geriatrician, an eldercare lawyer, and a financial advisor. (Review chapter 2 for details.)

It is important to build a meaningful relationship with our primary doctor. He needs to be made aware of all significant changes in our loved one's behavior. He also needs to be informed of any additions or changes in the medicines and dosages prescribed by other doctors. It is advisable therefore to keep careful behavior and medicine logs. These logs as well as written questions for the doctor should be taken to each regularly scheduled appointment to enhance the care of our loved one.

THE FAMILY NETWORK: POSITIVE SUPPORT (OR THE LACK THEREOF)

Alzheimer's is a disease that affects every member of the family. We may be the spouse of the loved one with AD, a sibling, or an adult child. We may be a grandchild, niece, or nephew. We may be a devoted in-law. All of us are gradually losing a loved one, an important person in our lives. Each family member will discover that he or she has a role to play in caregiving, whether it be helping with the care of the loved one or caring for the caregiver.

Family members provide the strongest link in the caregiver's support system. The family should meet regularly. As the disease progresses, the needs of the loved one and the caregiver change. The caregiver will need additional help, more respite. Family members should adjust their roles as caregiving becomes more difficult and more demanding. The ideal family works as a team.

In-town family members have no end of roles to play along the Alzheimer's journey. We suggest that during regular meetings, the family can determine how better to aid the primary caregiver as the disease progresses and the care needs change. Transportation, holiday gatherings, shopping trips, medical care for the person with AD, and respite for the caregiver are issues that will need refinement many times in the course of the disease.

If we happen to be an out-of-town family member, unable to attend the regular family meetings, our role may be to listen carefully when we have telephone conversations with our loved ones and the caregivers. We may be able to offer valuable advice in addition to emotional support.

Sarah, caregiver for her husband, Bob, tells of the weekly calls she received from her sister-in-law, who lives four hundred miles away. "My sister-in-law, Mary, called me every Saturday at the same time, 10:15 AM. She knew that by then I had Bob dressed and breakfast was over. We shared some of the small events of the week and I kept Mary up to date on Bob's condition. Sometimes her 'distant vision' enabled her to give me advice that really worked. Mary always had a joke for me. She knew how important it was for me to laugh. One Saturday she told me how much she wished she could come and help me. (Mary has a physical condition that precludes travel.) I replied, 'Mary, I don't know how I would manage without your calls. They are what I look forward to all week. Hearing your voice gives me such a lift and I know you will make me laugh.'"

Sharon had a different story to tell. After college she moved across the continent to begin a new life away from her clingy parents. When she discovered that her dad had Alzheimer's disease, she was torn; she didn't want to give up her life on the coast. She feared that if she went back home, even for a visit, she would be trapped and would never escape. "I was awash with guilt," Sharon confessed, "until I found out Mom was having difficulty paying for daycare. I saw a way I could help. I send her a check every month. And, you know, I think it's changing my relationship with my mother, just a bit. We're more like equals now. Why, I might even like to go back for a visit."

Dick lives three hours from his sister, Jan, a full-time caregiver for their dad with AD. He spends one weekend a month relieving her. Jan admits that without Dick's help, she doesn't know how long she would be able to continue.

Out-of-town caregivers can play important roles in the Alzheimer's journey. Mary, Sharon, and Dick found theirs. You can too.

We have referred to the family as a team of individuals working together to help the caregiver and the AD patient. However, the caregiver's family members may be scattered all over the globe, and the ones nearby may still reside in "Denial Land." If our family members are reluctant to offer help, we caregivers can build up resentment and anger that cause damage to our bodies. To prevent these stressful emotions we need to be realistic about the help our family members may be willing or able to provide. We also need to ask ourselves, "Am I giving the world the impression that I am handling my job as a caregiver with such success that I don't need any help?" If this is true, no one may ever offer to help.

We need to ask for help. We need to be specific: "I need someone to stay with Dad two evenings next month. I want to attend a support-group meeting and I want to go to the movies." Or, "What weekend next month can you care for Mother while I get away?" In-town siblings may respond to the first request. Out-of-town siblings may be able to answer the second call for help.

Sometimes the help we want so much isn't forthcoming. We must be careful that we do not let negative responses from a family member cause us to react with anger and resentment.

Evelyn remembers Roberta, a dear lady in one of her support groups who tried so hard to get her sister to help her occasionally with the care of their mother with AD. Roberta shared the difficulties she was having, the pain she was feeling. It was obvious that anger and resentment were about to bubble over, affecting her whole life. "My sister agreed to care for Mother from Saturday morning until Sunday noon," Roberta told us at that first meeting. "I planned a little getaway with a friend. I felt like a kid going on a holiday. Just overnight would be such a treat. My sister called Friday afternoon. She couldn't commit herself to the weekend—'something had come up.' She hung up before I could protest. I cried. I really cried. That was how disappointed I was."

At another meeting Roberta shared a different story. Her sister had finally taken their mother for the day. "She came for her on Saturday morning just before noon. I'd had Mother ready and waiting since ten when my sister had promised to come. So Mother was upset when I helped her into the car, and so was I. When my sister dropped her off (and that's what she did, at 5 PM sharp), she was full of complaints about what Mother had done all afternoon. She had bothered the children and kept her from her gardening. That's what my sister does: She either promises to look after Mother and at the last minute, after I've made plans, she cancels. Or, if she does take her, she does nothing but complain for days. Because I'm not married with children, she thinks I have nothing important to do when I'm not working. She has no idea how hard it is to juggle my job with Mother's care. I couldn't manage without adult daycare. It would be nice if my sister would appreciate what I do."

After the support group ended that day, Evelyn took Roberta aside to talk privately. Roberta admitted she was consumed (her word) with anger that was affecting her job performance, as well as the way she was treating her mother. She was afraid she would get sick because of the stress she was experiencing. Evelyn was able to get Roberta to admit that things had to change, and she had to be the one to change. She had no control over her sister. She did have control over her own actions and reactions. Evelyn suggested that a good way to start this change would be to stop asking her sister for help. Evelyn explained, "When you ask your sister for help, she tells you all the reasons she is too busy: children's school and sports games, her part-time job, a husband who wants her home on the weekends. When you prod her, she offers limited help. When she cancels at the last minute, you are hurt, angry, and feel unappreciated. When she does care for your mother, she complains bitterly about how her schedule was upset and how difficult your mother was. Do you really benefit from this kind of help? No! It really is no help at all.

"You resent the way your sister treats you. She causes you to become angry and feel diminished. This is the source of your anger. Do not let this continue. Promise yourself that not only will you no longer ask for her help, but that you will no longer want nor expect it. This attitude will place you in control. You need not react to her negative behavior. Treat your sister kindly, but change your relationship."

Roberta listened carefully but said little. Evelyn could not ascertain Roberta's reaction to the advice she had given. Roberta did not return to the support group the next month, or the next. Evelyn was afraid she had spoken too forcefully, hurting Roberta's already damaged feelings. Well, when Roberta appeared at the next group meeting, Evelyn was truly relieved. She thought, "She's back. Maybe I didn't scare her away."

Roberta explained to the group, "I've been so busy at work lately, I had to cut back on my outside activities. But you all need to know how much better I feel. I took Evelyn's advice and stopped asking or expecting my sister to help me. You can't believe how things have changed. I'm losing my anger. I am also realizing how my sister was feeling. She resented me, all the time I was resenting her behavior. When I asked for her help, she didn't want to give it. Then she felt guilty and was angry with me for making her feel guilty."

We wondered how Roberta had discovered this. She told us, "After about a month of not being asked to help, my sister seemed to relax when we were together. I realized that for the first time in ages I wasn't acting in an angry mode around her. One day it just all came out—how I felt, how she felt. We hugged. I felt cleansed of my resentment."

Roberta went on to explain, "My sister isn't offering her help yet. But because I don't expect it, our relationship is no longer adversarial. I can't tell you how much healthier I feel."

That was Roberta's last visit to the support group. Evelyn never found out if the sister was ever able to help with her mother's care. She likes to think that it did happen. Evelyn wasn't surprised that Roberta stopped coming to the meetings. She had received the much-needed help, and was now moving on.

We can hope that all of our family members would work as a team, but it might not always happen. There are many family members like Roberta's sister. They are caught up in their own busy lives. They are afraid if they once participate in even minimal caregiving, they will never be free of it. If these family members are not pressured into caregiving activities, there is a chance that eventually they might want to be part of the team. We must not harbor anger and resentment. We saw how that almost made Roberta ill.

William told the support group another familiar story—a story of greed. His wife's mother with AD was living with them. They had two teenagers who were quite helpful, doing chores around the house and occasionally staying with their grandmother while their parents had a night out. William and his wife, Julie, thought they had the caregiving situation under control. Julie decided she could return to work on a part-time basis. She had researched adult daycare facilities in their area and found one with an excellent activity director and a compassionate social worker. The daycare center even provided transportation. While Julie worked three days a week, her mother was in daycare. After three weeks in daycare, mother seemed happier than before; she was sleeping better because she was more active during the day. What could be wrong with this picture?

William told us, "Roger. He's what is wrong. I would never have believed he would have behaved this way. He has never been my favorite, but I didn't think he could be so selfish. What a jerk! Roger is married to Julie's sister, Joanne. When he discovered how much money we were spending on Mom's care he was angry. When he discovered that we planned to increase Mom's time at daycare to five days a week, he went ballistic. You see, we're spending Mom's money on daycare. We really can't afford to use our money, particularly with college costs around the corner. Roger tells us we are spending Joanne's inheritance. It was bad enough when we were spending the money for three days. 'Five days are just too much,' he says.

"Joanne says little. I can't tell whether she agrees with Roger or just doesn't want to get involved. I know she doesn't want to spoil her good relationship with Julie. Joanne does try to help out with her mother's care, but she lives an hour away. That's probably good. I've made up my mind about one thing. Roger's not going to have a say in how we care for Mom.

"I tell Julie we're lucky that she's the one with the power of attorney. We're trying hard not to let Roger upset us. But, can you imagine someone being that greedy?"

Roger is an example of a family member who needs to be handled carefully. In this case he is an in-law. He could well have been a blood relative. Some uncooperative family members criticize actions the rest of the family has taken, disagree with the diagnosis, or don't like the doctor. Because they did not have a part in many of the decisions, they take no responsibility for carrying them out.

These family members may be reacting to myriad negative emotions that have built up over the years. Their causes may be readily identified or buried too deep to sort out. There may have been intense sibling rivalry, a vying for parental approval, a need for peer acceptance and appreciation, or a need to dominate. The list could go on. The result is resentment and a feeling of separation from the family. It is important that these members do not interfere with the family's resolve to provide the best care for their loved one with AD. They may be annoying, but they must not be given a stage on which to perform.

We, the caregivers, will focus our attention on the family members who give us positive support. We will be thankful for their presence in our lives, and we must tell them so.

For the caregiver with limited family support, the next part of our support system takes on great importance.

FRIENDS AND NEIGHBORS

One night, Evelyn was trying to pull herself together after a particularly difficult day of caregiving. She was close to "losing it." She knew she needed a quick fix of positive thinking. She asked herself, "How many friends or neighbors would you feel comfortable calling at 2 AM? You ask for help and they respond with one question: 'Is your front door unlocked?'" Evelyn counted nine people she knew she could count on for help in the middle of the night. That was enough of a morale boost to send her to bed with a happy, grateful heart.

This account needs a little clarification. Two factors played a large role in the high number of helpful friends and neighbors. Evelyn and her husband lived in a town-house community with neighbors close by. However, equally important is the fact that, after the formal diagnosis, Evelyn never tried to hide her husband's illness. Her friends and neighbors knew of his gradual decline and difficult behaviors. They knew she needed help, offered it often, and gave it without her asking.

We know not everyone is as fortunate as Evelyn. The point we are trying to make is: if you try to hide your loved one's illness and give the impression there is no need for help, it will not be offered. The girl who didn't want anyone to know that her father with the brilliant mind was losing his cognitive skills was putting a barrier between her father and his friends. The husband who feared their friends would exclude them from social events if they knew of his wife's mental decline was paving the way for the very exclusion he feared.

In order for our friends and neighbors to be a part of our support system, we need to be open and honest about our loved one's disease early on in its progression. Friends will then understand the gradual decline in our loved one's social behavior. They will become more comfortable including him in group activities.

It is when we try to hide the disease (it really can't be hidden for long) that friends may exclude Dad or Mom. They do not understand the different behaviors and may feel uncomfortable. It is sad if this happens. With an open relationship, friends may be willing to take Mom for a ride or walk with Dad in the afternoon. If Mom or Dad lives alone, neighbors may be glad to keep an eye out for any strange behaviors. They may be willing to include them in an occasional trip to the store.

TIPS FOR FOSTERING GOOD RELATIONS
WITH YOUR FRIENDS

- Invite your friends for afternoon tea or dessert and coffee after dinner. Give your friends an opportunity to be with your loved one in a social setting.
- Find a friend to be a telephone buddy.
- Ask for help, but don't expect too much.
- Be specific as to your needs, e.g., "Can you watch TV with Dad while I run an errand?"
- Accept refusals graciously.
- Accept an invitation that includes your loved one.
- Leave before he gets tired.
- Write thank-you notes.
- Be grateful for every friend and helpful neighbor.

GAIN KNOWLEDGE TO UNDERSTAND THE DISEASE

A good way to start caring for yourself is to learn as much as you can about the disease. Call the Alzheimer's Association Helpline number for specific information. They will answer your call 24/7. They can tell you how to connect with your local chapter. The association prides itself on the individual service it provides for everyone who calls. Information can be given over the phone and informative brochures and fact sheets can be mailed to you. (See the appendix.)

Learning about the disease helps us appreciate what is happening to our loved one. It keeps us from overestimating his abilities and thus expecting too much of him. We learn that it is the disease that causes the challenging behaviors. Our loved one is not trying to be difficult. Understanding the four As, the symptoms of dementia, helps us better understand the challenging behaviors.

Amnesia

Most people understand amnesia, or memory loss, as a symptom and recognize it when a loved one can't remember, in the afternoon, what he did that morning. But we should also realize that because our loved one has short-term memory loss, he cannot with any certainty tell us whether he had his lunch or took his morning medicine. For a while he may be able to keep track of the day (marking it off on the calendar—looking at the morning paper), fix small meals, and even manage his medicines, using the weekly boxes divided into days as well as AM and PM. (Even people without AD find these med boxes a great help.) If our loved one is living alone, he needs careful monitoring. The caregiver needs to begin to plan for alternative care when our loved one can no longer safely live alone.

Aphasia

The loss of communication skills is also easy to recognize when our loved one finds it increasingly difficult to find the right words to express herself, often using inappropriate words and phrases. What we may miss, however, is that our loved one not only can't retrieve the correct words and phrases, but also that she no longer understands the meanings of many words (usually nouns) the caregiver is using (see chapter 5). Without the complete understanding of aphasia, we may become frustrated, upset, or angry when our loved one ignores our simple requests or directions. If we don't realize she doesn't understand what is being said, our anger can cause our loved one to respond in anger. Now we are both upset. Proper knowledge could have avoided this unpleasant event.

Agnosia

The inability to receive and understand sensory input is a symptom that comes later in the disease and is not understood by the uninformed. Our loved one could be in the kitchen next to a pot of beans. The pot has boiled dry; the beans are burning. The caregiver, in another room, finally smells the burning odor and rushes into the kitchen. Not understanding why his mother with AD has not turned off the stove, he may respond with anger.

Or, for instance, the doorbell rings. Dad hears it but the sound has no meaning for him. He does not answer the door.

The fork next to the plate is no longer recognized as a utensil used for eating. The list goes on as the caregiver gradually takes over the tasks of feeding, bathing, dressing, shaving, teeth brushing, etc. With prompting, the AD patient may be able to help with these tasks for a while. This cooperative effort takes time and much patience on the part of the caregiver. These tasks take longer to accomplish and cannot be rushed. The AD patient cannot perform these usual tasks and may resent being helped—a real Catch-22. Agnosia is the hardest symptom to deal with. The informed caregiver knows what to expect. He may be angry at the disease, but he understands that his loved one is not to blame.

Apraxia

The inability to perform coordinated movements, including the ones we consider automatic. Although this symptom appears much later in the disease, the AD patient gives hints of its onset when he exhibits difficulty getting out of a chair or a bed, and walks with an unsteady gait.

Having a better understanding of the disease makes us better caregivers. Make that call to the Alzheimer's Association. Ask for help with your specific problem. Use the Internet for additional information. We are learning, we are acting, and we are losing our denial. It is time for the next piece of our support network.

SUPPORT GROUPS

The Alzheimer's Association can help you find a support group. Unless you live in an isolated area, you should have several from which to select. Visit a few and choose one that seems best suited to your needs. There may be groups for adult children or spouses in addition to those serving all caregivers.

Watch how denial can sneak in here!

- "I don't need a support group. I can manage by myself."
- "I don't want to listen to other people's problems. I have enough of my own to worry about."

- "A support group? Sounds like a great big pity party to me."
- "Why should I share my life with perfect strangers?"

Now listen to the voices of support-group advocates:

- "I could never have made it without my support group."
- "I learned so many good tips for caring for Mom. It saved my soul."
- "We laugh more in our group than we do anywhere else."
- "No one truly knows what it (the Alzheimer's journey) is like unless he is a caregiver himself."
- "I can be honest about my feelings. Everyone understands. I can vent some of my anger at the disease. The group validates my anger."
- "I feel loved. My support-group friends really care about me."

These are actual testimonials from support-group members who came from all walks of life. Evelyn was the facilitator of two support groups for ten years. She saw firsthand the help that was given and received, and the strong bonding that took place in a loving, accepting environment.

If you have decided not to try a support group, you may want to carefully rethink that decision.

The Support Group and Role Reversal

If we are caring for one of our parents with AD, we are experiencing what is called "role reversal." We are losing one who was the mainstay of our life. We are giving advice when we are accustomed to receiving it. We are not comfortable being the one in control. Many emotions are causing us discomfort: fear, because we may be unequal in meeting the demands on our time and energy; guilt, because we don't really like our new responsibilities; anger, in response to our parent's anger when we exert our authority.

In a support group we discover that we are not alone. Others experience these disturbing emotions also. It is normal to feel fear, guilt, and anger. We learn how others are accepting their new role, adjusting their behavior, lessening their fear, banishing their guilt, and redirecting their anger to the disease. Out of their stories come ideas that we can use in our growing acceptance of role reversal.

The Support Group and Role Addition

If we are caring for our spouse with AD, we are discovering that we are into "role addition." Not only are we performing all our previous jobs, but also we have assumed the jobs that were our spouse's responsibilities. We are doing double duty. Our support-group members can reassure us that we can "get by with a little help from our friends."

We need the name of the car mechanic, plumber, electrician, roof repairer, etc. We need the beauty parlor number, the tax accountant's number. We are learning to shave, blow-dry hair, wash and shop for clothes, balance the checkbook, plan and shop for the meals we are learning to cook. We are overwhelmed. We need help! Our support-group buddies can help us work through the denial, voiced in the phrase, "We'll manage, we always have."

Because we were brought up to assume our own responsibilities, we think it's just short of shameful not to manage our own affairs. As a lady from Philadelphia of excellent upbringing said, after moving to Texas in the early 1800s, "A true lady kills her own snakes." Whatever our gender, we should admit we need help killing our snakes! It is not shameful to ask for help. It is smart to do so.

A support group can help us find ways to help our caregiving parent if he or she is in denial or refuses needed help. In a support-group environment, we are with others who are experiencing or who have experienced the very problems we face. They understand our feelings. They can share the ways they successfully dealt with trying situations and seemingly unsolvable problems. Through it all, they will help us activate our sense of humor and even make us laugh. Gradually we will find that we are the one helping others.

RESPITE OPPORTUNITIES

Respite: a short interval of rest or relief (Webster).

This word is music to the ears of the tired, harried caregiver. It is an absolute necessity for all caregivers. Remember the mantra: *I can't take care of you unless I take care of myself.*

One of the best respite programs available for caregivers is adult daycare. We believe so strongly in the program that we have devoted a whole chapter (see chapter 8) to explain why it is so beneficial to both caregivers and loved ones. We address the denial arguments and help you move into the acceptance mode.

Another source of respite is from an in-home caregiver. Your local Alzheimer's chapter should have a list of reputable home-healthcare agencies in your area. Also, you might find a well-recommended home caregiver by networking with your friends and neighbors, or at your church, synagogue, or mosque.

In-home caregivers provide a variety of services: companionship, meal preparation, light housekeeping, and transportation to doctors. There are aides who help with bathing, dressing, feeding, and making sure medications are taken properly.

It is important to hire someone who is familiar with Alzheimer's disease and the various behaviors that are associated with the disease. This is true whether we are hiring someone from an agency or someone we have met through our networking.

But we authors can hear the voice of denial loud and clear:

- "I won't let a stranger take care of my wife."
- "We can't afford to pay someone to care for Mom."
- "No one can take care of Dad the way I can."
- "I don't need anyone to help me care for my husband. Yes, I'm tired, but I can manage."
- "My sister and I check on Mom every day. She's doing fine."

We agree that not every family will need to hire someone to assist with caregiving in the home. Some caregivers will truly benefit from outside help; it can be a godsend. Outside help can provide the needed care to keep Mother, who lives alone, in her own home for a longer time. Checking on Mother may be sufficient until we begin to wonder if she is eating properly or taking her meds. Our loved ones with AD often neglect personal hygiene. And remember, she can tell us anything, but do we really know what is happening in her home when we aren't there? Someone to be with Mother on a regular schedule will give her the assistance she needs.

Bathing is one of the ADLs ("activities of daily living"—including dressing, eating, bathing, toileting, and mobility) that can cause the care-giver the greatest problem. This is a multilayered task that eventually becomes impossible for people with Alzheimer's to perform on their own. To people who are confused, this is an overwhelming task. Just the undressing is difficult. They are afraid of the water. They are afraid of falling. They feel their modesty is being violated. Caregivers step in to help and are met with strong resistance. The person with AD often simply refuses to participate.

The following amusing story shows how one family solved the bathing problem by using the help of an agency caregiver. (Remember the denial statement above: "No one can take care of Dad the way I can.")

Brian and his sister shared the caregiving of their father with AD. Brian's sister cared for him during the day. Brian and his wife picked him up after work and cared for him until the next morning. It was an arrange-ment that was working well for everyone. "Dad was happy," Brian reported. "All was going smoothly until Dad absolutely refused to bathe. We tried everything. I hoped he would be willing to shower if we did it together. No deal."

A friend suggested that Brian hire an agency caregiver, experienced in giving baths. Often a third party has success because she is not emotionally involved. Brian hired a woman experienced in bathing reluctant AD patients. Brian told us, "After interviewing Delia, I knew she would be suc-cessful. She was so kind and reassuring. We arranged for her to meet us at my sister's house the next morning. That night I told my dad about this woman who gave wonderful baths. She knew how to give the best back rubs in the world. I raved about her; how she had made me feel like a new man after one of her baths. Dad was very impressed. The next morning, on the way to my sister's house, I told Dad again what a wonderful bath he was about to experience. Dad was interested to hear how I had enjoyed her bath-giving talents.

"When we arrived at my sister's house, Delia was waiting for us. She succeeded in charming my dad right away. They went into my sister's spa-cious bathroom while the rest of us waited in the sitting room. When Dad and Delia joined us a while later, Dad had a big smile on his face. He looked at me and said, 'You were right Brian, she gives one terrific bath. Now it's your turn!'"

Brian still gets a laugh out of that story and remembers how relieved he was to have solved the bathing problem.

(As an aside—it is helpful to know that a daily bath is not necessary. The elderly tend to have dry skin, making daily bathing inadvisable.)

Mother needs time during the week to have a few hours of relaxation and entertainment, as Dad's care becomes truly a 24/7 responsibility. A rested caregiver is a better caregiver. If there are no family members to provide this care and Dad is not attending daycare, then getting help from an agency makes a lot of sense.

The argument "we can't afford it," becomes the ultimate excuse when we don't want to do something. Who can argue with that statement? No one can look inside our checkbook or wallet. If, however, we decide that help is a necessity and not a frill, we may be able to fit the cost into our budget. Family members can be a source of help. Investigate help through the local office on aging. The local Alzheimer's chapter may know of grant money available for respite care.

Once again, we are saying, "Ask for help."

Mention vacation to a caregiver and we may see an empty stare. He may be thinking, "Vacation? Take a vacation? You must be crazy. I can't leave my loved one. I don't need a vacation."

Evelyn would have responded the same way if someone had suggested she leave her husband with AD and go off for a good time. But Evelyn says, "Somewhere in my subconscious mind, that need for respite was strong. One night when the weight of winter was heavy on my heart, I blurted out to an empty living room, 'I want to go to Cancun!' Of course this was a ridiculous statement. I get sick in the sun, I never swim in the ocean, and I don't like hot weather. But at that moment I truly wanted to go to Cancun—I thought."

Evelyn's son Bruce lives an hour away by plane and is always ready to help. At that time his work was such that he could come without much advance notice. Bruce counseled her, "Mom, why don't you plan a long weekend in Bermuda? It's closer than Cancun. You can be there in three hours. I will come on a Thursday to take care of Dad. Just give me a couple of days' notice. Dad and I will have a great time together while you get a breather. I won't have to return until Tuesday."

Now Evelyn had this nice long weekend to look forward to. She bought a Bermuda outfit. A friend gave her a Bermuda travel book. Another friend gave her maps and brochures of all the places she had visited. Evelyn pored over the maps, chose her hotel, and found a wonderful hiking route. She even had an offer from another friend: "Evelyn, if you go in February, I can go with you."

Evelyn never went. She never made the trip to Bermuda. But you see, she could have. Her spirits brightened just thinking about the blue ocean, the pink buildings, the shopping, the good restaurants, and the getting away. She could go any time she chose. *And because she could, she didn't need to anymore.*

Let's look at the family that needs a vacation. They are caring for Mother, who has Alzheimer's and is not able to go with them. There is no other family member to care for her. This is the time to look into facilities that provide temporary respite. Many assisted living facilities offer respite for a weekend or longer.

The first time Karen decided her family needed time away from Mom, she found an assisted living facility that would provide care for a weekend. It had pleasant rooms, a helpful staff, and organized activities. Karen's mother did not want to go. She didn't put up much of a fuss, but her body language and "harrumphs" made it clear to everyone that she was into the martyr role. Karen confessed, "I felt awful. I changed my mind a hundred times, but I knew my husband and two kids needed a break. I felt guilty. I cried, but I did it. The family had a great weekend. I wasn't sure what to expect when we picked up Mother, but I never would have dreamed I'd find her in such a happy mood."

Karen explained that it was easier the next time they went away for a weekend. She didn't feel so guilty. Mother still didn't want to go to the assisted living facility, but she wasn't as unpleasant about it as before. By the third time, Karen said, "It was so easy. We knew how well they cared for Mother, and Mother was happy to go." Karen's family experienced the real bonus later. When they could no longer care for Mother at home, they moved her into the assisted living center that she already knew. It was an easy transition.

Karen told us, "It was hard watching Mother decline. When we knew we had to move her to assisted living permanently, I was really upset. What made it bearable was knowing that Mom was going to live in a place she knew, with people she knew taking care of her. It's strange how it all worked out. What I didn't want to do—hated to do at first—turned out to be what was best for us all in the long run. Those respite weekends eased Mom gradually into assisted living. We visit all the time. I'm pleased with her care."

When we need help beyond that which our family and friends can offer, we must not let our denial keep us from considering professional respite care. We may never use an in-home-care provider or an assisted living center as a source of respite, but it is important to know that we can. This help is available.

Chapter Five

"Honey, Please Hand Me the Broom"
Developing Communication Skills

One sees clearly only with the heart.

—Antoine de St-Exupéry

REALIZATION OF LANGUAGE LOSS CAN BE SHOCKING

W e share smiles; we hug; we laugh together. We frown and glare and stamp our feet. We cry tears of joy and tears of sorrow; we clap our hands in appreciation and acceptance. Then there are the high fives and thumbs up or down. There are so many nonverbal signals we use that effectively communicate ideas and feelings. Look at the face of a baby who cannot talk, or the body of a teenager who won't, and we learn more than words could ever tell.

Words, however, are the true coins of communication. Without them we feel poor. In our denial, wishful thinking, or ignorance, we may not know or be willing to accept the fact that language loss is a part of Alzheimer's disease. The sudden realization that our loved one cannot find the right words to speak, nor can he or she understand our words, may be overwhelming. We have learned to live with the memory loss. But language loss—oh no! Another layer of the denial onion to peel back.

Evelyn felt she had been blindsided when she first realized her husband had significant language loss (another example of how well the loved one with AD can compensate for his losses). She hadn't expected this loss, wasn't prepared for it, and could find no one to ease her into acceptance. Evelyn remembers some very dark days.

It was a cool October day. Bare sycamore branches were silhouetted against the pewter sky. The maple branches were still covered by leaves that seemed to fall in singles or pairs when not hastened by a mild breeze.

Raking leaves would be an enjoyable, productive activity for some weeks to come. Evelyn rested on her rake and watched John, busy pulling leaves out of the bushes one at a time. He was happily engrossed in his job. With a feeling of comfort, knowing this productive job for John would stretch into the following month, Evelyn got back to work.

In a few minutes she called to John, "Honey, please hand me the broom."

John looked up with a totally blank expression on his face. Evelyn knew at once that he had no idea what she wanted. Using her hands in a sweeping motion, she said, "I need the thing you sweep with." Now, with a smile on his face, John handed Evelyn the broom.

The feeling of comfort from a few moments before was replaced by a feeling of cold dread. What other words didn't he understand? Evelyn was shocked by the sudden discovery that her husband had a significant language loss. Had she not known it was a part of the disease, or had she refused to believe that it would ever happen to him?

Once Evelyn accepted the reality that John was losing language skills, she needed to place herself in a learning mode.

Just as action can help us out of avoidance, denial, and despair, so can knowledge. In this chapter, we authors share with you real communication situations that may resonate with your own experiences. We also offer realistic techniques that not only improve communication but also improve your attitude toward the language loss. By remembering the way we communicate in a nonverbal fashion and by adopting suggestions that will help in your own circumstances, you will be better able to accept this rocky part of the Alzheimer's journey and to communicate more successfully with your loved one.

With diminishing communication skills, our loved one has a hard time successfully expressing feelings. This may lead to frustration and angry outbursts. A family member/caregiver without adequate knowledge may interpret this anger as an attack on him or her and respond in an inappropriate fashion. In this chapter, we help you understand some of the situations that can produce anger. When you trade your denial and avoidance for information, your reward will be an easier route through a troubling portion of the Alzheimer's journey.

Throughout the entire journey, we encourage you to share your smiles and hugs and to laugh together with your loved one whenever possible. Phyllis Diller describes a smile as a "curve that sets everything straight." A smile is, at the very least, the "gift that keeps on giving." A smile and a sense of humor reflected from caregiver to care-receiver and vice versa is a win-win situation.

Our loved one responds strongly to our mood. The smile on our face and the shared laugh become two of our most valuable communication techniques. Some may counter, "We can't laugh and smile all the time—this disease is too difficult to deal with." We respond, "Precisely—because it is so difficult to deal with, we must learn to smile more often. We must 'access mirth' to help us over the rough spots."

A COIN WITH TWO SIDES

As we try to communicate with our loved ones, we need to remember that there are two sides to the coin. On one side, we see the family members with AD who seem to have lost most of their verbal skills. We are never quite sure how much of the conversations they understand that go on around them. Because their verbal responses are few and seldom, some of us are uncomfortable in their presence. We don't know how to treat them. Should we include them in our conversations? How? Unfortunately, some of us choose to talk over and around our loved ones, in essence ignoring them. How sad!

On this same side of the coin, we find the family member who talks but makes little sense. How can we converse with someone who uses sentences and phrases that have no discernible meaning for us? In our discomfort, we may choose to avoid or ignore our loved one. Again, how sad!

Here are three important rules to remember when we are with our loved ones:

- Never discount what they can hear and understand.
- Never talk over or around them.
- Always include them in conversations even if they can't talk, or if their words make little sense.

There are countless stories about people who haven't spoken for some time or whose conversations make no sense, who will, without warning and often for no discernible reason, come out with a perfectly clear and appropriate response to a given situation.

PASSIVE PARTICIPATION

Then there are countless stories of nonverbal AD sufferers who passively participate in group conversations by focusing on the speaker, by demonstrating interest, and by laughing at the appropriate times. We can increase our loved one's passive participation by giving them the "best seats" (where they can easily see and hear everyone) and by deliberately including them in the conversation. If you are out with your husband, Bill, and everyone is talking about the local sports team, turn to him and remark, "Bill, remember the time we were in New York and watched our team cream the Yankees?" The conversation turns to politics and you might remind Bill what a loyal supporter he was every time Joe Doakes ran for office. Bill may simply nod his head or smile, but he knows he's been included.

Every afternoon Evelyn would take her husband, John, to social hour at the health center. They sat around a big table with other residents and family members. It was a time for soft drinks, chocolate chip cookies, and good fellowship. There was easy conversation and much laughter. Several regular visitors would often comment on John's behavior. They told Evelyn that his eyes never left her face when she was talking and that he laughed at all the appropriate times. John himself never spoke at these gatherings, but there was never any doubt of his genuine passive participation and true enjoyment during social hour.

Some of the residents at the table still had adequate verbal skills. It was heartwarming to watch them successfully interact with the few nonverbal residents. There was an abundance of love and acceptance around the table that eased the sorrow in all of their hearts.

What may be more difficult for us than having no conversation is responding properly to the non sequitur or the comment or question we don't understand. Evelyn learned the perfect solution to this problem from the Alzheimer's patients themselves.

RESPONDING TO THE NON SEQUITUR

Every Friday, Evelyn took her sister-in-law, Helen, to have her hair done. It was a pleasant twenty-minute ride in the country to the beauty parlor. Helen enjoyed the day, which included lunch, and if she was able, a bit of shopping. There was, however, one big problem. While they were in the car, Helen directed her many comments and questions to the passenger side window. With her almost deaf right ear, Evelyn could understand her sister-in-law only if Helen turned her head and spoke directly to her; otherwise, Evelyn could understand only a part of what she was hearing. Evelyn would ask Helen to repeat her question. Helen couldn't because she could not remember what she had just asked. Nor could she remember to direct her voice toward Evelyn. They were both frustrated. Evelyn tried so hard to understand Helen's words and Helen wanted so much to be understood.

Fortunately for both, Evelyn learned early on how to solve the problem. One morning at Helen's nursing home, she watched two women residents engaged in conversation. There was talking, laughter, and gesturing; their total enjoyment was evident. They were talking to each other in turn, responding to each other, laughing with each other. After several minutes they ended their encounter with a warm hug.

Evelyn knew both of those women well. They were delightful ladies. She enjoyed being with them when she visited Helen. Not capable of completing a sentence that made much sense, they began a conversation with one idea and ended with a totally different one. How could they converse with each other in a conventional manner, exhibiting such enjoyment? The answer is obvious.

These ladies were acknowledging each other. They listened to each other and responded. We all need this kind of validation. We need to be able to express ourselves, to have someone listen and accept what we have said. For the person with AD, this acceptance and validation is hard to achieve in a world of words and cogent ideas.

These ladies had information to share. They understood what it was. They wouldn't have been able to communicate it to you and me, but how gratifying it was to be accepted and validated by a friendly housemate.

Let's get back to Helen in the car on the way to the beauty parlor. She made a comment. Evelyn heard the word *trees* and responded, "Yes, Helen, these trees are much taller than last year." Helen made another comment. Evelyn heard nothing clearly, but responded, "I'm surprised the corn has grown so high this early." This worked beautifully! Helen was being acknowledged and Evelyn's frustration returned to a comfortable level.

THE OTHER SIDE OF THE COIN

Let's take a look!

Our loved ones have compensated for their losses for so long. They have learned when to smile and when to look as though they understand what is being said. They have kept their social skills, which are often among the last to be lost. They know the appropriate questions to ask: "How are the children?" "Have you had your vacation yet?" "I hope you have been keeping well." "I like your outfit. Is it new?"

Mother, who has kept her social graces as the disease progresses, can converse on the phone quite comfortably with her out-of-town children. This causes them to believe she is more capable than she is. The problem is that what she tells them about her daily life may or may not be true.

On this side of the coin, we see family members with AD with verbal skills that fool us into thinking they are far more capable than they really are.

Let's look at both sides of the coin:

Dad, on one side, who speaks only a few words, may understand much of what goes on around him. He is saddened when family members and friends ignore him. This may add to his depression or feed his anger. He feels alone and left out.

Mother, on the other side, with adequate verbal skills, fools her family into thinking she is still able to live alone. This can place her in an at-risk situation. Because Mother seems to be more capable than she really is, she may not receive the care and support she needs. Mother may also feel alone and left out.

Remember: our loved ones may understand far more than we suspect; or we may be expecting them to understand far more than they are able.

TIPS FOR IMPROVING COMMUNICATIONS

- Talk slowly. People with AD take a long time to process information.
- Give one-step directions. If we say, "It's time to get out of bed, put on your slippers, and go to the bathroom to brush your teeth," our loved one may retain "brush your teeth" but lose the preceding steps. When he makes no move to get out of bed, it's because that direction has been forgotten.
- Point and gesture. For the preceding set of directions, you may need to gesture to show how to move the legs over the side of the bed. Point to the slippers.
- Repeat. Use different phrases and always use a patient, happy tone.
- Avoid pronouns. Do not say, "Put them on." Do say, "Put on your slippers." Do not say, "Let's go over there." Say, "Let's go through the door."
- Listen, acknowledge, and include them. Even when your loved ones cannot carry on an intelligible conversation, listen and acknowledge them. Include them in your conversations.
- Don't argue. Step into their reality; agree with them, comfort them; make them feel safe and loved.
- Don't say *no*. Whenever you say *no* you are intruding on their ever-diminishing area of control. Instead try to divert attention or offer alternative suggestions.
- Reminisce. Not, "Do you remember?" but "Remember when—thus and such?" Then you are doing the talking and someone who is confused is not frustrated by his memory loss. Use old photo albums to help both of you remember. As the disease progresses, your loved

one will identify with older pictures of himself, and sadly not know who that person in the mirror is.

UNDERSTANDING ANGER

While all family members in denial benefit from looking for underlying causes of anger, our harried caregiver may need this understanding the most. Because she is so tired, she might counter anger with even more anger, potentially creating an unplanned and undeserved catastrophic event.

Let's look at the following scenario to understand the cause of some outbursts of anger.

Mother is in the doctor's reception area with her caregiver. She has no idea where she is or why she is there. She is surrounded by strangers. Only her caregiver has a familiar face. A nurse dressed in street clothes approaches Mother, takes her hand, and asks her to come with her. The caregiver nods approval and Mother walks down the hall with the nurse to a small examining room where she is asked to remove her clothes. Not understanding what is happening, Mother forcefully refuses. The nurse, with many demands upon her time, tries to hasten the process, whereupon Mother lashes out with voice and fists in an effort to protect herself.

We are now dealing with a catastrophic reaction, which may cause the nurse to label this patient aggressive and difficult to manage. A repetition of this episode may result in a consideration of treating the aggression with medication. But is medication the answer?

What has caused this catastrophic event? Mother isn't being aggressive and difficult. *She is simply scared to death.* She is defending herself against an aggressive stranger who wants to remove her clothes! Wouldn't you do the same thing?

Now let's turn to the caregiver—the hardworking, loving daughter who would never intentionally hurt her mother. Her mother has always enjoyed going to visit the doctor. She liked looking at the magazines in the waiting room, chatting with the nurses, and joking with the doctor who looked so young and handsome. Mother had never behaved like this before. What happened?

It has been three months since Mother last visited the doctor. She no longer remembers the office, the nurse, or the procedure in the examining room. We can only hope that her daughter will recognize this change and realize that Mother's angry, aggressive behavior was caused by fear. That being so, she does not deserve the "aggressive patient" label.

Mother needs to be walked one step at a time through her visit to the doctor. Her daughter needs to be with her in the examining room to assure her she is safe. Her daughter needs to remember to give directions one at a time, with gestures if necessary.

Angry outbursts from our loved one are often caused by fear or extreme frustration. By removing the cause of the fear and eliminating these frustrating events, we can save our loved one and ourselves from the exhausting effects of an anger episode.

ANOTHER CAUSE OF ANGRY BEHAVIOR

Aunt Susie was a perfect lady. She spoke correct English, devoid of any slang expressions; she never uttered unpleasant comments, let alone swear words. She wore a hat and gloves when going to town and was a formidable presence to the storekeeper who treated her with the deference and respect such a lady deserved. Aunt Susie developed dementia. After a few years she moved to an assisted living facility run by a pretty young woman with a delightful disposition. One day she approached Aunt Susie, intending to invite her to tea in the day room. Before the director could issue her invitation, Aunt Susie cried out in a vitriolic tone, "Get away from me. Don't touch me, you son-of-a-bitch!" Aunt Susie's niece, sitting nearby, was in complete shock when she heard these words. She could not believe it was her aunt speaking.

Fortunately the director of the assisted living facility later explained to the niece that as the Alzheimer's disease had progressed in her aunt, parts of her brain had been damaged. Aunt Susie had lost her inhibitions. She no longer had the control to prevent the angry outburst the niece had witnessed.

We have all learned how to control our behavior and to conform to expected standards. We might, in the privacy of our bedrooms, utter a swear word after stubbing our toe, but never in front of anyone. (Well, hardly ever!) We might jump up and down in the kiddy pool, recklessly splashing water as we cry in delight with our two-year-old child, a behavior we would never exhibit with our friends in the adult pool.

Aunt Susie no longer monitored her behavior; she just did "what came naturally." She was angry enough to swear, and so she did. Freud would say, "Her id is loose and running rampant." When self-awareness is gone and there is brain damage due to the plaques and tangles of Alzheimer's disease, inhibitions disappear. Persons with AD may act very much as they always have, or, depending on where the damage occurs, they may become totally different people, doing things they have never done before.

The director explained something else to the niece. Aunt Susie had been angry with her earlier in the day when she had kept her from going out on the shopping tour. The residents take turns for that trip. It was not Aunt Susie's turn. Although she couldn't remember the earlier morning event that caused her anger, the emotion could be remembered far into the afternoon.

Memory of the emotion stays while the memory of the causative event disappears. What a wonderful incentive for promoting a safe, happy environment, with lots of smiles and good humor—the gift that keeps on giving.

UNRESOLVED ANGER

Irene had worked hard all of her adult years. She had held responsible jobs in banks and in a prestigious auditing firm where first she was the office manager and then executive secretary to one of the partners. Her husband was selfish, demanding, and often away on business. They had no children. Irene had few friends and a limited social life because of her husband's unpredictable presence. She felt unappreciated at work and at home. She never voiced any displeasure or dissatisfaction with a life that was out of balance: too much work, too little pleasure, too little emotional support. She never expressed any anger or resentment toward the people who benefited from her generosity and charity, and who took and took and gave so little in return. Irene was doing what she had been taught—work hard and make the best of the hand you have been dealt.

Irene developed Alzheimer's disease. She had a philosophical attitude toward her condition. She would say, "I can't do anything about it. I might as well accept it." As the disease progressed, Irene moved from assisted living to a nursing home where her condition gradually worsened. With her inhibitions gone, she began to experience many unexplained outbursts of anger. She would spit out nasty words to anyone in her presence. Her face took on a contorted expression of displeasure. No one was able to jolly her out of her almost constant anger. No diversion could separate her from her nearly obsessive angry behaviors.

Irene had one loyal friend, Marie, who was a frequent visitor. One afternoon Marie wheeled Irene out to the patients' garden where they could see beautiful flowers and listen to the songbirds. A soft summer breeze cooled their faces as they sipped iced tea. Surely, Marie thought, this environment would soothe and calm Irene. It did not. Irene yelled at the aide serving the tea. In a loud, nasty tone she told one resident to "shut up" and another to "go home." These were sweet ladies sitting quietly, enjoying the summer afternoon.

At this moment, Marie had an epiphany. Of course Irene was angry. She had every right to be angry. She had half a lifetime of bottled-up anger. Now that she had lost her inhibitions, the anger was coming out. Instead of trying to soothe Irene, Marie knew she needed to validate her anger. "Irene, it's all right to be angry. With whom are you angry?"

Irene looked at Marie and said firmly, "Him! I'm angry with him."

Marie said calmly, "I don't wonder, Irene. Let's be angry with him together. I'm going to stamp my feet to show how angry I am. You stamp your feet, too."

Irene began stamping her feet. She held Marie's hand while they stamped together. In a few minutes they stopped. For the first time that afternoon Irene looked calm, even peaceful. For the moment her anger was gone. Indeed, Marie had used the right treatment—validate Irene's anger; tell her it was all right to be angry; and then help her to release some of that angry energy.

In subsequent visits, Marie was often able to appease Irene's anger by validating it.

How often we, who consider ourselves "well," need to have our feelings acknowledged. This is no less true for our loved ones. When they hurt, it doesn't help for someone to tell them that everything is all right. What may help is for someone to accept their feelings, showing sympathy and concern.

In Irene's case, there was a reasonable, underlying cause for the suppressed anger that was bubbling to the surface. Sometimes excessive noise or confusion surrounding our loved one may cause an outburst of anger. She communicates her displeasure and discomfort in a display of anger. It may help us discover the cause of the anger if we ask ourselves what happened before the outburst. Was there an environmental factor that could have caused it? What time of day did she demonstrate the anger? Was she being rushed? Is there a pattern? Was she "sundowning"? (See appendix.)

The answer to these questions may help us understand the "why" of the anger and how to make proper adjustments. A change in routine, fatigue, an upset caregiver, a frustrating task, or any physical ailment: each may produce a feeling of anger that our loved one will act out. Our loved ones may not be able to tell us that they don't feel well. They may have a headache, a stomachache, or a toothache but cannot communicate this information. They may not be able to tell the location of the discomfort. A urinary tract infection can also cause behavior changes. It may be time for a visit to the doctor.

Often we cannot find a reasonable answer to the "why" of the anger. It is helpful to remember that our loved one may be scared, frustrated, bewildered, or disturbed. He lacks the ability to communicate these feelings verbally and may not remember or understand what caused these emotions in the first place.

The caregiver needs to respond with quantities of love and patience. "Where," you ask, "is all that patience coming from?" You will see more about our prescription, "Patience, Perspective, Humor," in the next chapter. Then take a good look at chapters 4 and 9 on caring for the caregiver.

Chapter Six

"She's Just Pushing My Buttons"
Challenging Behaviors

Many fears are born of fatigue and loneliness.

—Max Ehrmann

INCONSISTENT BEHAVIORS

Yesterday morning, Mother awoke before anyone else. She dressed herself without help. She didn't make any mistakes. This morning she was back to her "helpless" state and couldn't do a thing without me. When it suits her purpose, she can manage to dress herself just fine. I swear, she's just pushing my buttons. She always did know how to get a rise out of me. Enjoyed it too! This was such a busy morning. Why did she have to be so difficult today?

How hard it is to work through layers of family emotions when dealing with dementia! Daughter, who does not understand Alzheimer's, believes Mother is deliberately trying to upset her to make things difficult, particularly because this was her pattern of behavior before the onset of dementia.

Daughter never resolved the feelings of resentment and anger toward her mother. These emotions are laced with love and guilt. Now, Mother's behavior seems to match her former patterns. Being in denial, Daughter cannot believe it is the disease that deserves the anger, not Mother.

Daughter is another good example of a tired, harried caregiver. We hope she will read further in this chapter to get a different perspective of her mother's disease. We validate her anger when it is directed at the disease and not at Mother. Mother is sick. She has a disease and the disease has a name.

Inconsistency in behavior is confusing and often feeds the sense of denial. Caregivers and family members need to remind themselves continually that their loved one has a disease. This disease causes her to exhibit unusual behavioral symptoms. While one may often see a logical reason for illogical behavior, we cannot always understand why Mother could dress herself one day and not the next.

Individuals with AD may exhibit behaviors that differ from day to day. Fatigue, infection, frustration, or a sense of well-being might trigger unexpected behaviors. Our loved one is doing the best she can in any given moment. And that moment is all she can remember.

Caregivers need to use to their advantage the knowledge that behaviors change with the emotional and physical environment. When dealing with a problem (dressing, eating, bathing, etc.), what didn't work today may work tomorrow. The opposite is true, also. Caregivers have to "go with the flow," trying not to let difficult behaviors cause them to exhibit anger.

In the morning, we tried to get Mother to eat her breakfast. She wouldn't touch it and, after more coaxing, let out a yell and threw it on the floor. She had forgotten how to use the utensils to eat, and her temper got the better of her.

Our loved one is not trying to "push our buttons" or cause us grief when she exhibits different, aggressive, or annoying behaviors. These are responses to stimuli that elicit negative behavior. And these behaviors are part of the disease. Our loved one can become frustrated when she is unable to perform a simple task. She may be frightened when she doesn't understand a simple direction. She may be overwhelmed when the directions, the task, or the caregiver's impatience demands a response that is totally beyond her abilities.

THE NEED FOR ONE-STEP DIRECTIONS

It is important that we remind ourselves that as the disease progresses, the symptoms intensify. Mother's memory loss is now so great that she cannot respond to multistep directions.

"Pick up your spoon and eat your cereal, Mother." Mother may retain only the words *your cereal*, and she may not know the meaning of the word *cereal*. We see amnesia (memory loss) and aphasia (the inability to understand words) working together. Mother cannot follow our directions because she does not remember them and she does not understand all of our words.

We need to use one-step directions, use hand signals, and repeat if necessary.

Mother is beginning to lose her ability to process sensory stimuli. She doesn't pick up the spoon to eat her cereal, because today she does not know the spoon's use. She may need cueing to get started. Put the spoon in her hand and help her carry the cereal to her mouth. Once started, she may be able to continue by herself. It is a little like putting the phonograph needle in the right groove. Once there, it can play the tune.

PROCESSING AUDITORY STIMULI

Let's look at what can happen when an auditory stimulus is not properly processed.

The telephone rings. Mother is close to the phone. Daughter, in the next room, expecting Mother to answer it, gets upset when the phone keeps ringing. Mother must first identify that the noise is a ringing sound. Then she must remember what causes that sound—doorbell, television, or telephone. "Oh, it's the telephone. Now, where is the phone? Oh yes, there it is. Now what do I do with it? I pick a piece of it up—which piece? Now what? One part goes to my ear. Which part? Now what do I do? It will be easier if I just leave it alone."

Later in the disease there will be no connection at all in her mind between the ringing sound and the telephone. They are separate entities.

Now, Daughter in the other room becomes upset because Mother doesn't answer the phone. Her anger and frustration impact on Mother, who cannot understand why Daughter is so angry. She wants to please. She tries so hard. Mother's reaction to Daughter's anger may be tears, or verbally or physically aggressive behavior.

STOP!

Is there a way out of this dilemma?

Step back—let's take a long look at ourselves.

DENIAL PREVENTS UNDERSTANDING

We get angry when we expect behaviors from our loved one that she is no longer able to give us. This anger is fed by the state of denial that keeps us from fully understanding the extent of her cognitive loss.

Now let's take a long look at our loved one.

We can understand why AD is called the "hidden disease." Mother looks great. Her hair is done every week. Her clothes are clean and coordinated (thanks to a conscientious caregiver). She still has her social graces. She can still perform most of her ADLs (activities of daily living—see appendix). We want to believe she is all right. But she is not all right. She is sick. She has a disease—and the disease has a name—and that name is Alzheimer's.

Only when we admit that Mother is not OK can we begin to make things easier for her and for ourselves.

It's all right to be angry, but the anger should be directed at the disease and not at our loved one. Mother may not have been the easiest person to live with when she was well, but she doesn't deserve our anger now because she is sick. When we look at the reasons for our anger we realize, that in addition to our frustration over difficult behaviors, unexpected behaviors, and unwanted behaviors, we are dealing with a disease that demands so much of our time and energy. We become frustrated and fatigued.

All too often we don't receive the help and support we feel is due to us from family members and friends.

Sometimes we doubt our own ability to deal with the disease and wonder: "Why me? Can I do this?"

Often buried, because it causes us shame, is the sense of loss. We've lost our "normal" lives and want to go back to the way things were—before. We don't like it here in Alzheimer's Land. We want OUT!

There may not be an "out," but we may find a way "around"; a different way, a different approach. Many events in our lives are beyond our control. *But we can control the way we deal with these events.*

In our sense of denial we may feel trapped. Can we believe there is a way to control—not the disease—but ourselves? Can we learn a more successful way to deal with the problems caused by AD?

A POWERFUL PRESCRIPTION FOR SANE CAREGIVING: PATIENCE, PERSPECTIVE, HUMOR

We know how important it is to maintain a level of patience. With it we can handle problems with greater ease; difficult situations don't overwhelm us. Our loved one responds favorably to the pleasant tone of voice that patience provides.

When we lose our patience it may be because we are bone tired, but more often it is because we have lost a proper perspective and with it our sense of humor. Patience is a by-product of perspective and humor.

The following true story helps to illustrate this:

When Evelyn was preparing for Christmas, one of the most important decorating tasks was installing lights in every window in the house. When her husband was able, this was always his job. The candles were dusted, the lights tested, and the proper extension cords were attached and plugged in—often behind heavy pieces of furniture. John made it seem like an easy task. Eventually this became one more job that Evelyn had to take on because of the progression of his AD. For her, this was not easy. It took most of the time that John was in daycare for her to decorate. As she was driving him home, Evelyn began planning the way she would get John to help her light the candles. It would be a good activity to fill the time before dinner. Once in the house she began to show John how to turn the light on, lower the shade, and partially close the draperies. It was important that only the lower center pane remain uncovered. Evelyn was looking forward to walking outside in the early evening dusk to see how pretty the house looked "all lighted up."

Well, it was not to be. Evelyn did not realize how confusing the whole operation was for John. Nothing went the way she planned. If the light was on, John turned it off. If it was off, he turned it on. If the shades were pulled down, he raised them. If the shades were raised, he lowered them. Closed draperies he opened—opened ones he closed. John was becoming agitated.

Every window that Evelyn fixed, John "unfixed." She was getting more and more upset. This was an important Christmas decoration, almost as important as a beautifully trimmed tree. She had worked so hard all day. A knot of anger formed in Evelyn's stomach as tears welled in her eyes.

Then, miraculously, a wonderful feeling overcame her anger. She began to see what was happening from a different perspective. It made her laugh. She imagined people out on the sidewalk in front of her house looking at shades up, shades down, lights on, lights off, draperies open, draperies closed, wondering, "What is going on in that house?" She imagined how Lucille Ball could have turned this debacle into a half-hour sitcom and she laughed some more.

Evelyn quickly got all the draperies closed. John became calm. The next day she packed up the lights and the extension cords, and put them back in the cupboard in the basement where they remain to this day.

A proper perspective opened the door to humor, and patience returned. Again, patience is definitely a by-product of proper perspective and humor.

This being true, we need first to examine *perspective*.

We may have no control over the disease, but we do have control over how we deal with it. Our attitude is of prime importance. Are we victims or are we conquerors? We are not helpless. We win when we accept. Controlling our response to negative events takes practice. We need to say, "I will try." It helps to have some key phrases to remind us to stay on firm footing and not slip into the modes of anger, frustration, and helplessness.

Does It Really Matter?

When Mother chooses to wear an orange sweater that clashes horribly with a purple skirt, when Dad wants to wear his slippers to bed, when our spouse stirs coffee with a knife in the restaurant, does it really matter? Probably not.

We need to choose our battles. We need to help Mother change her Depends; forget the sweater. Dad needs to brush his teeth; forget the slippers. Our spouse is having such a good time in the restaurant. We don't want to spoil it by shaming her.

Denial, not worked through, becomes our enemy when caring for a loved one with AD because it keeps us from recognizing reality and making appropriate and necessary changes in our own behavior. As the disease progresses and our loved one's capabilities diminish, we are continually required to reassess how we should be treating our loved one. Evelyn remembers learning that what had seemed important in the past no longer mattered.

Helen, Evelyn's sister-in-law with AD, was a meticulous dresser. She bought beautiful clothes that were altered to fit perfectly. Her closet always held clothes never worn, in readiness for any fancy occasion that required a special outfit. When Evelyn became Helen's caregiver, she wanted her always to look as attractive as she had when she was well. Evelyn bought her becoming dresses that were easy to put on. At her nursing home, everyone declared Helen the best-dressed resident on her floor. This made Evelyn feel good, even though it was uncertain if Helen still cared.

It became harder and harder for the aides to pull on Helen's panty hose. But Evelyn insisted. She wanted her dressed in the same fashion as before. Evelyn is not sure when or why she came to her senses. The day she brought a supply of knee-highs to take the place of panty hose, Evelyn had shed denial to look at reality. When Evelyn bought the first supply of white wool socks, she remembered how in the past she had looked at the residents who wore them with a bit of sympathy. Didn't their family members care how they looked? Of course they did, but they also cared about keeping cold feet warm.

Evelyn had a much easier time going from linen napkins in a fancy restaurant to piles of paper napkins and tasty finger food in the mall's food court. Helen's dining abilities declined, as did her ability to wait patiently for the food to be served. Waiting for the check presented another problem. Helen couldn't understand why she couldn't leave as soon as the meal was eaten.

When Evelyn geared their experiences to Helen's ability, they had happy times because Helen was always successful.

As Alzheimer's progresses we need to change our expectations and adapt our activities to the present abilities of our loved one. We cannot continue to follow old patterns. We learn that what does matter is a happy, successful loved one.

As our perspective improves, it's amazing how many things "don't matter"!

Never Argue

In the early stages of the disease, it may be helpful to orient our loved one into our reality but, when the orientation turns into an argument, it is time to stop.

Mother looks out the window and sees the next-door neighbors working in the garden. She exclaims, "The Fosters didn't go to the ocean this weekend after all! I wonder why. They told me they were going."

Daughter answers, "No Mother, the Fosters weren't going to the ocean. The Smiths across the street are the ones who told you they were going to the ocean."

Mother, a bit upset, continues, "The Fosters told me they were going away, not the Smiths. I know who it was."

Time for a reminder: never argue!

Arguments can cause catastrophic reactions for our loved one and extreme frustration for the caregiver. Often times what was argued about *didn't really matter.*

Sometimes we find ourselves arguing about something that does matter. George found himself in this situation. But arguing achieved nothing but headaches and anger. His support-group buddies helped him find a way to solve his problem.

George told his story with pain in his voice. His friends listened carefully to see if they could help. George's wife, Alice, often awoke before he did and dressed by herself. This did not present a problem until Alice needed to wear Depends in the daytime as well as at night.

George would awaken to find his wife fully dressed, wearing her underpants instead of Depends. Getting Alice to change into the Depends before going to daycare had become such a battle that some days he chose to stay home with her.

"I don't know what to do. I can't stand the arguing and the struggle every morning."

After a moment of silence in the group, Jane spoke up and asked, "Does Alice keep her underpants in a certain place in her bureau?"

George answered, "Her lingerie drawer is so neat, with her underpants, bras, and slips stacked in separate piles."

Jane made a suggestion. "Get rid of all the underpants and put Depends in their place. See if that works."

George quickly exclaimed, "I can't do that!" He went on to explain that this was his wife's drawer. This was her underwear. He couldn't get rid of them. They were hers.

Several weeks later, the group met again. This time George had a success story. In desperation, he had followed Jane's suggestion. It worked. No more morning arguments over Depends versus underpants.

"But, Jane," he said, "it was so hard to throw Alice's underpants away."

In our denial we try hard to keep the life that "was." We refuse to admit that the life that "is" needs adjusting.

Evelyn tells the story of a simple adjustment that solved a problem and created a welcome chuckle.

Peter ate lunch at the table with Evelyn's husband, John, at the nursing facility's dementia day program. Peter was far more cognitively able than John, but John had better manual dexterity. This made John a "neater eater."

The lunch menu included soup, which was often the best part of the meal. Peter truly enjoyed the soup, even as he spilled much of it down his bib and onto his shirt. John was able to eat without spilling a drop, finishing his meal without a spot on his shirt.

Peter's wife, Vera, arrived every day at the end of the meal, greeting him with the same words, "Oh, look at you. You're such a mess. Why can't you eat carefully the way John does?" Whatever enjoyment the men had shared during lunch disappeared as Vera took off Peter's bib, wiped his face, and dabbed unsuccessfully at the spots on his shirt.

It didn't matter to Peter if he spilled his soup, but it did to Vera. She felt it was shameful to see her husband with a bib and food spilled down the front of his shirt. John was a reminder of how things used to be.

The remedy for this situation proved to be easy. Evelyn separated the juice from the solid part of Peter's soup, and directed him to drink the liquid and spoon the solid. No more spills. Peter got a chuckle from this procedure. "Vera would have a fit if she knew I was drinking my soup."

When we are out of denial we see more clearly the need to change expectations. We learn what does matter and what does not matter. We know that arguing with our loved one is counterproductive.

Rearranging Reality

As the disease progresses, we recognize that our loved one's reality is no longer our reality. Because we can no longer bring our loved one into our reality (we have stopped arguing), we must slip into his. This requires us to create false situations and tell lies in order to make our loved one comfortable and ease his fears. This is often called "creative lying" or "therapeutic lying." Because one of Evelyn's support-group members was so upset over the thought of telling deliberate lies, Evelyn came up with the term "rearranging reality." It is something most of us have done throughout our lives, consciously and unconsciously. Now we can rearrange reality to ease difficult situations. It benefits both the loved one with AD and the caregiver.

The following story involving Evelyn and her mother-in-law with AD shows one way rearranging reality worked:

"My mother-in-law wanted to 'go home' on a regular basis. I arrived at her apartment one afternoon and found her 'ready for the movers.' The twin mattresses were stripped of all linens and spreads. All light bulbs were removed from lamps and stored in bureau drawers. Drawers were also stuffed with towels, soap, toilet paper, and all knickknacks from the living room. All pictures and mirrors were off the walls and tied together. How this five-foot, one-hundred-pound woman accomplished all that alone, I'll never know. But there she was that afternoon, suitcase packed, pocketbook full of costume jewelry, two coats over her arm, ready to go. 'Where are the movers?' she asked me.

"In an instant I knew the role I had to play. 'Oh Mother,' I said, 'you won't believe what those movers have done! They have mixed up the dates. They just called and told me they can't be here until tomorrow.' I embellished my story a bit more, creating a group of movers on whom she and I could vent our anger. It was wonderful the way it worked. Mother directed her anger to the movers and I was her buddy as together we restored order to the apartment.

"Other times, when Mother wanted to 'go home,' I would assure her that it was too late, too rainy, or too cold that day. 'We will go tomorrow,' I would promise. 'We'll get an early start and bring a picnic lunch.' Then I would ask her questions about her mother, her home, and what she did as a child."

Often the desire to "go home" is reflective of a need for the security of home and the love of "Mother." Sometimes reminiscing and looking at old photo albums will relieve the homesick ache.

In addition to the desire to "go home," people with Alzheimer's disease have a need to be with dearly loved family members. They do not remember that their mother, spouse, or close sibling is dead. Dad may ask often, "Where is your mother? She should be home by now. I hope nothing has happened to her." We recognize his growing concern. We can tell Dad each time he asks for his wife that she died several years ago. Each time we tell him, he relives the sorrow he felt at her death. We know he will ask the same question over and over. Do we really want to inflict this pain again and again? Of course not.

Instead we rearrange reality. We give Dad a reasonable explanation for Mom's absence. She can be at a bridge game, shopping with friends, attending a meeting—whatever fits with her previous activities. We assure Dad that Mom is safely engaged and will be home soon.

Mother may be upset because her sister, Mary, hasn't called or written lately. She's angry with Mary, but also worried about her. We can tell Mother that Mary died many years ago. Mother reacts to this information with anger. She insists that Mary is alive. "You don't know what you are talking about. Mary is not dead. You are just trying to upset me!"

We can try to reason with Mother with no success. This becomes a "never argue" situation. Rearranging reality solves the problem. We tell Mother that her sister is on a vacation trip and will be home soon.

Our rule of thumb is this: Tell any lie that will soothe, comfort, or reassure your loved one as long as it will do no harm to anyone else. And, if you want to bring a bit of healing humor to the situation, remind yourself that you don't have to remember your lie—your loved one won't.

Rearranging reality is a technique we need to learn early and use often. It can smooth the rough spots and prevent arguing.

When she learned it was time to paint the house, Brad's wife, Joyce, went willingly to the healthcare center. This was Brad's way of rearranging reality. The health center placement was necessary. Their house was not being painted. Joyce was deathly allergic to paint fumes. Brad would take paint chips to the center whenever Joyce seemed impatient to return home. Together they would choose paint colors for bedrooms, den, kitchen. After several months Joyce was settled into the health center and did not ask to go home.

Paula looked forward to going to her church service every Sunday. One Wednesday morning she appeared for breakfast "dressed for church." No one was able to convince Paula it was Wednesday; not even newspapers, calendar, TV, radio—nothing worked. Paula's niece remembers what a dreadful time they had. She learned from her support-group friends how futile it is to argue when a creative lie could solve the problem. They assured the niece that the family should have stepped into Paula's reality and agreed it was Sunday. Then a reasonable story could be invented: the heating or cooling system in the church was not working; the clergyman was out of town and missed his plane; her church service was postponed until evening because of these difficulties.

One small humorous aside before leaving "Rearranging Reality." At John's healthcare facility, Evelyn learned the exception to the rule "never tell your loved one that his or her spouse is dead." Mrs. Taylor was an extremely attractive woman of about eighty-five years. She came to America from Scotland when she was in her teens, but she never lost her Scottish burr. It was still possible to orient Mrs. Taylor to time and place. Every morning Mrs. Taylor would ask Evelyn, "Where am I? What am I doing here? How long have I been here?"

When Mrs. Taylor felt reasonably comfortable with the answers, she would ask *the* question, "Where is my husband?"

Mrs. Taylor's daughter had told Evelyn how to answer this question. "Mrs. Taylor, don't you remember? Your husband died a number of years ago."

Mrs. Taylor would smile and, in her delightful Scottish burr, reply, "Oh, thank goodness! I thought he might be out with another woman."

Never Say No

We must try to remember that our loved one is losing control of his life. It is not easy for him to accept that all decisions are made for him and not with him. If we are careful, we can preserve his dignity by giving him small choices and avoid his anger by redirecting it instead of saying *no*.

When Dad wants to go for a walk without wearing a jacket on a cool afternoon, it may be easier to get him to comply with our wishes if we give him a choice. Instead of saying, "You can't go out without a coat," we should ask, "Dad, would you rather wear your leather jacket or your denim jacket? Which one do you think looks better with your pants?" As we present two jackets, we give him a choice rather than a command. If he still chooses to leave the house without a jacket, we should just bring it along. When he finds out how cold it is outdoors, he will welcome our casual comment, "Oh, Dad, it's much colder than we thought. I'll bet you'd like to slip on this jacket."

Mother causes a mild disaster every time she goes into the kitchen to "help get dinner." You try to remove her diplomatically but usually end up with a cross tone of voice as you tell her, "No, Mother, I don't need any help. Please go into the living room." This may put tears in Mother's eyes and guilt in your heart. As guilt builds up it forms a hard core of resentment that feeds the anger you feel against Mother, the disease, your unappreciative siblings, and your absent husband and children. It's time to have your own private conniption!

Can we intervene in this progression of events and emotions? We can try. Instead of saying no to Mother, let's try to redirect her attention to a pile of napkins (paper or cloth) that you have conveniently stored in the dining room. "Mother, these napkins need to be folded. Would you mind sitting here at the table and helping me out?" Mother needs to help. She needs to be wanted, not shunted aside. A careful examination of minor kitchen and meal-connected activities may provide tasks (however much unneeded) that Mother can perform. She will feel productive and connected to the task of meal preparation that was hers for so long.

In a sincere attempt to improve our perspective and thus our caregiving skills, we need to remind ourselves continually of these key caregiving phrases: Does It Really Matter? Never Argue—Rearrange Reality. Never Say *No.*

Will all of these techniques work all the time? Of course not. Will we remember to apply these ideas to the appropriate troubling episode? Not always. But every time we don't argue, for example, and it works, we will begin to feel better about ourselves as caregivers. We will realize that we are managing "in a positive fashion" the difficult behaviors this disease can provoke. Our perspective will improve. We will have more patience.

Introduce Humor

Now it is time to introduce humor into the equation.

Remember the story of Evelyn and John's Christmas lights? When Evelyn saw the humor in the situation and began to laugh, her knot of anger dissolved and was replaced by a proper perspective. Without humor, we become like the earth that receives no rain. It dries up and cracks.

Mark Twain tells us: "Humor is the great thing, the saving thing, after all. The minute it crops up, all our hardness yields, all our irritations and resentments slip away and a sunny spirit takes their place."

Henry Ward Beecher said: "A person without a sense of humor is like a wagon without springs—jolted by every pebble in the road."

A sense of humor acts like a shock absorber for caregivers and loved ones as they travel the Alzheimer's road with its pebbles, boulders, and unexpected twists and turns. As we caregivers develop our abilities to smile and laugh, we enrich the lives of our loved ones. How much better our loved one will feel when he or she sees a smile on our face instead of a frown.

Our loved ones are keenly aware of their caregivers' emotional states. They pick up on anger and internalize it. They become upset and may not know why. It is important to stay calm and to radiate love. Our loved ones depend upon us for their sense of security and well-being. If our behavior is out of control, how frightening it must be for our confused loved ones. If we lose our perspective and respond to their frustration with anger, we have robbed them of security and love. How different the results will be if we learn to smile. If we can laugh *with* our loved ones and laugh *at* ourselves we reduce our stress and improve our immune systems.

As we learn how to deal with, and more important, learn how to prevent difficult behaviors, we make our task of caregiving much easier. We owe it to ourselves to take that step out of denial and to adjust our perspective. We also owe it to ourselves and to our loved one with Alzheimer's to examine our attitude and to try a new approach.

Remember our key words:

- Patience
- Perspective
- Humor

Chapter Seven

"Dad's a Danger to Himself and Others" The Driving Dilemma

Take kindly the counsel of the years, gracefully surrendering the things of youth.

—Max Ehrmann

THE LOVE AFFAIR WITH OUR CAR

We have devoted a separate chapter to the "driving dilemma" because, indeed, for so many families the driving problem matches Webster's definition of the word *dilemma*: "a predicament that seemingly defies a satisfactory solution."

The "right" to drive. That ranks up there with the right to life, liberty, and the pursuit of happiness, doesn't it? We all remember as teenagers waiting for that piece of paper, the license that brings with it a true sense of control, mobility, and freedom. Many of us would willingly admit that our first love affair was with a Mustang, T-Bird, or VW. We remember the thrill of our first solo drive. Owning a car was the ultimate dream.

Most of us keep up that love affair with our car. Our sense of control continues as we go where we want, when we want. Our mobility expands. We drive to school and work; to the dentist and doctor; for a night on the town. We haul groceries, furniture, garden plants, the soccer team. We use the automobile for family vacations. What was once our teenage dream becomes a necessity.

It is no wonder then, that when advanced age and/or dementia call into question the ability of a loved one to drive safely, the family faces a dilemma. How can they determine when their loved one is no longer a safe driver? Then, how can they successfully move him permanently from the driver's seat to the passenger's seat without incurring his wrath and robbing him of his dignity? How will the family members manage to add their loved one's driving needs to their ever-growing list of responsibilities?

THE FAMILIAR VOICE OF DENIAL

There are no easy answers. Not knowing how to approach the problem, the family postpones positive action with an unspoken prayer that nothing bad will happen. It is denial that speaks out.

Listen for a familiar voice:

"I don't want to be the one to tell Mother she can't drive. She'd put me in my place fast. No one ever tells her what to do."

"Dad only drives to the doctor's office and church. Certainly nothing can happen on back roads."

"My husband will get angry. He equates power and independence with driving."

"What will I do if my husband can't drive? I haven't been behind the wheel in years. I've forgotten how to drive. We would be completely dependent on our children. We only go to the store and the doctor's office."

"Mom only drives for necessary errands. If I have to add them to my already overloaded schedule, I will be swamped."

"Dad will only drive in his familiar neighborhood; what harm will that cause? It will save me so much time and effort."

"Look at how difficult it will be if my husband can't drive? Who will take over all of the driving chores? We will be stuck in our house."

Can we recognize ourselves in any of these scenarios? Can we hear our own denial and fear?

Our denial may be prompted by a desire to maintain the status quo, which is so comfortable and convenient.

We have good reason for building a false sense of security to avoid anger from Mom and/or Dad. After all, we are children trying to tell our parents what to do. We want to avoid our parents' anger at any cost. We are not comfortable with this role reversal. Mom and Dad have always been the ones with good advice for us. Now we will be expecting them to abdicate their position of authority as we advise *them*. We feel guilty and afraid as we consider dealing with this issue of control and independence. We may decide to wait, wait a little longer before we address the driving problem.

Denial fosters delay.

When denial takes over during the driving dilemma, it becomes our true enemy. It can place a person with dementia behind the wheel of a car and keep him there long after he has shown signs of cognitive loss and diminished driving and problem-solving abilities. A potential disaster is on the road every time he drives the car. While getting lost or meeting unsavory characters are real dangers, a car accident involving precious lives may loom as the unforgivable, preventable disaster.

A CAREFUL LOOK AT REALITY

No one wants to face that unspeakable horror, so let's put denial aside and look carefully at reality.

A person diagnosed with Alzheimer's may be able to drive successfully in the early stages of the disease. Short trips around home or driving with a passenger to provide guidance may be quite appropriate. Those drivers with long years of successful driving experience, before the onset of AD, will probably be able to continue driving safely longer than those drivers with less experience. However, at some point all people with AD have to stop driving. Because of the uncertain progression of the disease, the family must remain alert to determine when it is time to stop.

A safe driver must have the ability to make correct, quick decisions. He must absorb countless cues that determine speed, lane choice, and defensive driving techniques. A person with Alzheimer's loses these skills in an inconsistent manner. Today his driving may be within acceptable limits while tomorrow he may demonstrate serious impairment. This factor alone can feed the family's denial, prompting the statement: "Dad is just having a bad day."

UNSAFE BEHAVIORS CONSISTENT WITH DEMENTIA

Some of the unsafe behaviors consistent with dementia include:

- Not seeing or paying attention to traffic signals, crosswalks, or pedestrians
- Getting lost in "home territory"
- Driving in the wrong lane
- Unsafe passing procedures
- Delayed reaction time
- Difficulty making quick stops
- Inadequate defensive maneuvers
- Backing into cars in a parking lot
- Becoming tired and confused
- Mistaking the accelerator for the brake pedal

POSSIBLE CONSEQUENCES OF UNSAFE DRIVING

Some of these behaviors may cause inconvenience, dents in the car, or small, no-injury accidents. But if we set denial aside and look squarely at reality, we will understand that unsafe driving coupled with the confusion of AD presents the distinct possibility of serious consequences, such as:

- The driver gets lost, wanders from the car into a wooded or uninhabited area.
- The lost driver suffers a medical (e.g., a diabetic) emergency and is without the medication to alleviate the problem.
- An accident occurs involving serious injury.
- An accident occurs causing death.

Can we afford to stay in denial? No! These consequences have, unfortunately, happened to others. We must not let them continue to happen.

Our denial has been fed by fear. We have feared our spouse's or parent's anger. We have feared change. We have feared inconvenience. We dread the thought of additional tasks and responsibilities. Is any one of these fears or inconveniences equal to the fear or consequences of our family member causing the death of another driver? This is a heavy responsibility to contemplate.

Alzheimer's changes the lives of the person with the disease and of all his family members. We may have no control over these changes, but *how we react to these changes is always our choice*. If we have taken a good look at the driving reality, we know we must change our attitude and move into action.

We hope we have captured your attention.

A FAMILY GATHERING TO AGREE ON SPECIFIC ACTIONS

Now we are going to offer some practical suggestions and tips that will help you through this difficult time. Exactly how you handle the driving situation will depend upon your own particular circumstances. You may want to try several approaches to solve this problem.

First, it is advisable to have one of those family gatherings described in chapter 3. This time have the meeting without your loved one present. All the other family members should meet to create and present a unified front. It is advisable to have a leader of the group and a recorder. It is crucial for the family to agree on the following actions:

- Treat the family member with AD with respect. His feelings will always be acknowledged kindly.
- Allow him to drive as long as it is safe for him to do so.
- Wean him slowly from the more difficult driving situations.
- Research and plan alternate means of transportation.
- Monitor his driving.
- Stop his driving when he is no longer a safe driver.
- Choose the best way to stop his driving.

HOW TO IMPLEMENT THE ACTION PLAN

Decide who will be best suited to carry out each of the following actions:

- Breaking the news to your loved one of the family's collective thoughts
- Researching alternate transportation
- Monitoring driving
- Stopping his driving

Gradual Weaning—Plant the Idea Early

Surrendering one's right to drive is a difficult and emotional experience. Because termination of the driving priviledge becomes an absolute necessity as the disease progresses, *the topic should be introduced early on while the confused driver still has decision-making abilities.* Call upon his sense of fairness when you explain that eventually it will be unsafe for him to drive.

At your family gathering you have chosen one or two members who know that even in the face of anger they will be calm, loving, and understanding when they talk about the need to eventually give up driving. In the conversation with your loved one, introduce the idea that for everyone the time will come when driving will not be safe. Include the fact that people, as they age, have slower reaction time and poorer vision, and eventually they stop driving.

Remember that your loved one has short-term memory loss. The conversation about driving cessation needs to take place more than once, and always in a kind, gentle manner. The message may not be received graciously. It may cause an angry outburst. Your response should reflect patience *and understanding* as you acknowledge his anger:

"Dad, I know you are angry. Of course you don't like the idea of giving up driving. I would feel the same way. We can talk about it later. But for now, think about letting someone else do the night driving."

The next time you bring up the driving subject you need to assure Dad that he will have transportation to all of his important activities when his driving days are over. The family member who has researched the transportation possibilities can produce a tentative plan including family members, friends, taxis, or senior-ride programs. Having the information at hand will help Dad see that being told he will be provided with needed rides was not a hollow promise.

Carefully, gently, plant the seed. His driving days will eventually end. For now encourage him to let others drive:

- At night
- During inclement weather
- During rush hour
- On highways

A gradual weaning from full-time driving may make it easier for him to give up driving completely.

Assessing Driving Ability

There are several ways to assess driving ability:

- Be a passenger, alert to any infractions of safe driving rules or delayed reaction time.
- Look for signs of fatigue, confusion, or poor judgment.
- Follow the driver without his knowledge. Pay strict attention to all his driving moves.
- Examine the car for small dents or nicks.
- Note times when errands take much longer than usual. Did the driver lose his way?
- Keep a written record of all the above—with dates.

In addition to assessing ability, you must also factor in the growing confusion, memory loss, and problem-solving difficulties you notice when your family member is not behind the wheel. These behaviors can be exacerbated under the stress of driving. And driving today can be a stressful experience.

Evelyn was jolted abruptly out of her denial when her son returned home from the library one day and without any preamble announced, "You have to take the car away from Grandmother before she kills everyone in town!" Drake had been walking to the library when his grandmother spotted him on the sidewalk and offered him a ride. As he told about his mile drive with her, he explained why he felt that he and everyone else in town was in danger with Grandmother behind the wheel.

Drake had correctly assessed his grandmother's driving ability. Evelyn and her husband acted quickly. They took the car. After a gentle explanation, saving Grandmother's feelings as much as possible, they tried to preserve her dignity and promised her they would chauffeur her wherever she wanted to go. Oh, there was anger—a lot of it. And resentment, accompanied by an "I'll get even with you" attitude. She succeeded in this by asking to be taken places she didn't want to go at times that were extremely inconvenient.

After about a month the anger and resentment vanished. Grandmother rather enjoyed being chauffeured around. She stopped her inconvenient requests. It was worth dealing with all of the unpleasant behavior knowing that "everyone in town" would be safe from Grandmother's dangerous driving. That was a successful scenario because Evelyn and her husband knew what had to be done and did not let Grandmother's tears and anger stop them or compromise their position. They "bit the bullet" and were willing to experience any unpleasant behaviors to assure no driving accident would occur. (It is important to note that no one else needed to use Grandmother's car.)

Evelyn's family was fortunate that their son's correct assessment of Grandmother's driving prevented a possible disaster. However, how much easier it would have been for them all if they had not let denial cloud their vision and had gently prepared her for what was to come.

Slowly weaning a family member from full-time driving may help soften the actual event. Start with nighttime driving. Older people often have a difficult time with night vision and the glare of oncoming headlights, and are glad to let others do the driving. Your loved one may actually be relieved to let someone else do the driving during rush hour or during a rainstorm but won't admit it.

IT IS TIME TO STOP—WHAT DO WE DO NOW?

You've planted the seed, you have tried gradual weaning, and you've reminded your loved one of lawsuits that could result from an accident, or at the very least a rate hike on his car insurance. You gently but firmly tell him it's now time to stop driving. But he is adamant with his decision to continue driving. What do you do?

There are many different scenarios. Each family's experience is unique. You may have to use several techniques to solve the driving dilemma.

The first and most important thing you must do is stick to your decision. It is time. *Your loved one is not able to make this decision. You must.* Though it may cause unpleasant, difficult behaviors, you must not abdicate your responsibility. (Reread the possible adverse consequences.)

Remove the Car and License

You may decide to have the car do a "disappearing act" by selling it or keeping it at another family member's home. If she cannot see her car she may not ask to drive it. Taking the car worked for Evelyn because she was available to provide all desired transportation. But remember, Grandmother was not happy. She was angry, made a big fuss, and initially caused great inconvenience to the family. However, bearing the inconvenience was doable. And it may work for you. Remember, also, to explain how much money will be saved due to the cost of insurance, repairs, the high cost of gas. That might resonate!

When the vehicle is actually removed from sight, there is a possible downside that should be considered. Your loved one, not seeing her car in its usual spot, may decide it has been stolen and call the police. Or a more enterprising and able person, knowing her car has been taken from her, may find a way to purchase a new or used car. (This has been done!) For that reason it is wise to take possession of her license, too.

Disable the Car

Having a disabling switch installed in the car is another tactic to try. If the car is to be used by other family members, they must be taught how to use the switch.

You guessed it—there is a possible downside to this tactic also. If your loved one happens to be adept at car repairs, he may be able to fix the car. If not, he may decide to call AAA to come and start the car. (Now that's creative thinking still at work!)

Ask the Doctor for Help

Your doctor can play a key role in solving the driving problem. Share your concerns with him or her. Put in writing the poor driving behaviors that family members have recorded, as well as specific examples of confusion, memory loss, and poor decision making that can affect his driving ability. After reading this report the doctor may be willing to advise your loved one that it is time to stop driving. Ask the doctor to write this directive on a pre-scription pad. The prescription including the words "no driving at any time" can be used whenever needed to remind the family member that the doctor has made this decision and it must be adhered to. But what if the doctor decides that the doctor/patient relationship will be irrevocably harmed if he becomes the agent forcing his patient to stop driving? He may be willing to recommend that his patient go to a facility that conducts driving assessments, preferably the state motor vehicle administration. If he does not pass the test, his license will be immediately revoked. An independent driving school does not have the power to revoke a license. It can only make a recommendation.

The State Motor Vehicle Administration

The state motor vehicle administration (SMVA) may have a program to assist you. In many states a letter from a physician describing the impairment of your family member will begin a process that includes screening tests to determine driving fitness. The physician is granted immunity for a letter written in "good faith"—thus preserving the good doctor/patient relationship. Check with your Alzheimer's Association or the SMVA to determine the regulations in your state that may help you. Please note that a family member or friend/neighbor may also write to the SMVA describing pertinent behavior with the same guarantee of confidentiality that a doctor enjoys.

ABOUT THOSE CAR KEYS!

We have mentioned the importance of taking your loved one's license so he cannot purchase another car or drive someone else's car. But what about the keys?! We recommend that you replace the current car keys with keys from a former car. Possessing car keys may help maintain his dignity even if he never uses them.

Evelyn would always ask her husband before leaving the house, "Honey, do you have your keys?" He would finger them in his pocket as they walked out the door. Evelyn would do the driving, but in her husband's mind he still had the potential for driving—by having his own keys.

A BRIEF REVIEW

Let's have a quick review.

Although your loved one may still be able to drive, the family must face the unfortunate fact that *eventually all people with AD must stop driving.* Because the results of driving with the impairments of AD can be so severe and are preventable, *family members must push denial aside and face reality.*

- A family meeting will help get all members on the same page, working together. In unity there is strength. Assign each member a role in the process. *Never abdicate your responsibility to make the decision to stop your loved one from driving.*
- Monitor driving ability. Assess competency and record observations.
- Factor in confusion, memory loss, and ability to make responsible decisions.
- Broach the subject of driving *early in the disease process when the family member is still able to make rational decisions and understand reasonable arguments.*
- Gradually wean your loved one *from driving by having him give over the responsibility during difficult times—at night, during inclement weather, etc.*
- Be supportive, patient, and understanding, *knowing that this is a difficult time for your loved one.* Avoid arguments.
- Validate the anger *that may be expressed. Do not respond with anger.*
- Use a variety of techniques.
- Create alternative transportation plans.

- Do not let anything stop you *from carrying out your decision that your loved one must stop driving.*
- Understand that, although what you are doing may be difficult, it must be done.
- Overcome your denial early *to make the process easier.*

Some people with dementia are ready to give up their driving and are relieved when family members make the decision for them. Some expressions of anger are attempts to maintain control, to save face, or to keep things "the way they have always been." This is why the family's reaction, attitude, and behavior are so important. Never argue, or show anger, but divert attention, validate feelings, and give choices in other areas. The family must maintain its resolve at the same time it maintains the loved one's dignity. It is a fine line to walk.

Know that what you are doing is your best and only choice. You are practicing "tough love."

Chapter Eight

"The Lifesaver for Both Caregiver and Loved One" The Daycare Decision

People seldom see the halting and painful steps by which the most insignificant success is achieved.

—Anne Sullivan

THE POSITIVE VALUE OF DAYCARE

Mental, physical, and social stimulation are three important aspects of Alzheimer's care. However, there comes a time in the development of the disease when the usual activities of a social and recreational nature are less appropriate for our family member. She may still be reading, but understanding and remembering little. Rules for card games are forgotten, crossword puzzles are ignored, board games become impossible. Social functions are difficult, if not painful, for our loved one. Imagine holding your own in conversations all evening when you cannot remember what your companions are discussing! At first, your social graces, which are among the last of the skills you lose, will carry you for ten or twenty minutes. Then the strain begins to show.

Evelyn knows this well. Her husband remarked after several social occasions, "I tried so hard." Her heart ached for him.

Often, because social activities are so stressful, our loved one will begin to decline invitations. As the disease progresses the familiar becomes their safety. The home with the caregiver becomes a safe haven. Some people with AD resist the unknown (anything beyond the front door) so strongly, that they refuse to go out of the house.

For many of us who have been on the Alzheimer's journey, adult day-care has been the livesaver for both caregiver and loved one.

Adult daycare centers provide a structured therapeutic program in a safe, nurturing environment. Activities are designed to be failure free, meeting the cognitive needs of each participant. Activities are varied: word games, current events, crafts, cooking, gardening, dancing, outings, and in-house parties. Our loved one is socializing with others who share similar circumstances.

The center provides its participants with a well-balanced meal and snacks. Some of the available services may include bathing, podiatry, hair styling or barbering, personal counseling, and transportation to medical appointments. Most centers also provide transportation to and from the facility each day. Hours vary in each center, but many have hours to accommodate working caregivers.

Centers usually require families to enroll their members for at least two days a week. This helps to establish a routine, which is increasingly more important as the disease progresses. This gives caregivers a break from their heavy responsibilities.

We caregivers now have two days a week to attend to necessary tasks and appointments. We must be sure to use some of this time for renewal and recreation. *Remember! We can't be good caregivers unless we take care of ourselves.*

ANSWERING THE DENIAL EXCUSES

All that being said, where is the problem? A structured, safe, productive environment for our loved one and two days (or more, if you choose) for us to use for ourselves. Sounds great.

Let's look at some of the excuses denial can create:

- "Our mother isn't ready for daycare."
- "All the people at daycare are old and far less able than my dad."
- "She won't get along with the people at daycare. They have nothing in common. She will refuse to go."
- "My husband was never very social. He won't fit into that environment."
- "I've taken care of my wife for fifty years and have done a darn good job. Now that she really needs me, I'm not going to turn her over to strangers."

Let's look at each of these excuses. The first two are the ones heard most often on helplines. "My loved one isn't ready. She is far more able than anyone she would meet at daycare." In some cases, this may be true, but more often we have let our denial take over. One of our biggest mistakes is underestimating the cognitive loss of our loved one and overestimating her abilities. It is more comfortable to believe that our loved one is more able than she really is. Her high-level social skills may be fooling us. Entrance to daycare marks the public admission that our loved one is no longer a highly functioning adult.

Are we somewhat ashamed? It's natural, if we are.

If it is AD, our loved one has a disease, a disease with no known cause and no known cure. Our emotions must include compassion and love, not shame. We should admire the courage our loved one displays each day, as he or she struggles to perform the simplest of tasks. Again, we must not let the stigma attached to mental illness, still prevalent in our culture, cloud our vision. This is a disease of the brain, involving severe physical changes.

No, it is not shame we feel. It is grief.

This step in the care of our loved one forces us to admit our loss. The enormity of it may be overwhelming at first, for we realize that nothing will ever be the same again. Our loved one is gradually slipping away from us. We cannot change that. What we can change is our own attitude.

The next two excuses: "My loved one will have nothing in common with the participants" and "My loved one will not feel comfortable in such a social environment" are denials of the changes that have been occurring over a period of time. Our brilliant husband may no longer be able to converse on the intellectual level that he once did. Our nonsocial mother may be relieved and pleased to be in a social environment where her cognitive losses are commensurate with those of her companions.

One of the more comfortable excuses for not sending our loved one to daycare is: "I know he/she will refuse to go." This takes the responsibility out of our hands. We blame it on Mom or Dad. We forget that our loved one has lost the ability to make sound decisions. We know daycare is the right choice and we should act on that knowledge. This may be a good time to "rearrange reality." Because our loved one feels more secure in the safety of his home, he may initially reject the idea of daycare. Our own attitude is of prime importance. We must project our own enthusiasm for this venture. We can tell our loved ones they will be helpers at the center.

One man brought his briefcase each day. He was "going to work." Another man thought he was taking a part-time job after retiring. The staff gave him small jobs to do each day. One day he asked his son, "Where is my pay? I work every day and I never get paid." His son thought quickly and replied, "Dad, they use direct deposit. The money goes right into your bank account."

The staff at the daycare center will have many suggestions to help the caregiver and the family member with AD during the period of adjustment.

A common excuse from spouses who cannot bear to relinquish the care of their loved ones to "strangers" may be the most difficult to circumvent. On the one hand we may be looking at loving, caring relationships with decades of devotion. On the other hand the relationship may have had its rocky times and now the spouse has the opportunity to make up for past problems by being a supportive caregiver. The situation may necessitate some intervention on the part of the doctor or adult children. They need to persuade these spouses that daycare will enhance the life of their loved ones, while also helping the spouses maintain their own health. This combination will ensure their being able to continue to care for their loved ones. Sending them to daycare may be the "doctor's prescription," thereby relieving husbands or wives of the responsibility for the decision.

HOW TO MOVE OUT OF DENIAL AND INTO ACTION

To change our attitudes about adult daycare, we first have to see ourselves in a state of denial, then admit that our perceptions may be faulty because of our emotional tie to our loved one. *It isn't that our loved one isn't ready for daycare; we are not ready.* This is a time when action may help us.

We can look in the phone book for a list of adult daycare centers. We can call our local chapter of the Alzheimer's Association for specific information about centers near us.

It is a good idea to make appointments to visit the daycare centers in our area and to talk particularly with the social worker and the activities director. They can help us determine whether our loved one is appropriate for their center and calm our fears about the cognitive and age mix of participants. It is a good idea to carry a notebook in which to record the information we will need to help us decide which center is best for our loved one. (See below for tips on what to look for in an adult daycare center.)

If we are not already a member of a support group, this is the time to join one. Our local Alzheimer's chapter can provide a list of groups in our area. It is helpful to call the leader of the group, in advance, and tell her we want to find out as much as we can about adult daycare centers. If there are any doubtful or resistant members of the family constellation, they should go with us to the support-group meeting. At the meeting, we will find truly supportive people who will share with us their journey to "the daycare decision." Knowing what daycare center they chose and how helpful daycare has been for them might help us in our decision.

If the situation indicates, now is the time for a family council meeting to share all the information gleaned from visits to adult daycare centers and from the participants of the support group.

We should coordinate all information and decide:

- Which adult medical daycare will we choose?
- Which days will our family member attend?
- How will the cost be met? (Investigate financial aid available from the office on aging.)
- How will our family member be transported?

We should work with the daycare center to implement our decisions.

Now that our loved one is being well cared for, it is time for us, the caregivers, to take care of ourselves. We repeat the mantra: *I can't be a good caregiver unless I take care of myself.* We should try to use this time for R & R as well as a time to accomplish necessary tasks.

We must keep in mind that it will take a while for our loved one to adjust to daycare. During this settling-in time, he may resist going or even tell us he does not like the center. We should try not to let this upset us. We can call upon the staff at the center for suggestions to make the transition time easier for our loved one and ourselves. If we give it time, this new experience should become a comfortable routine for everyone involved.

A wonderful neighbor, Charlie, finally convinced Evelyn that her husband needed more physical and mental stimulation than he was receiving at home. It was spring. Evelyn had planned garden chores and daily walks for John's physical activities. She bought easy jigsaw puzzles and rented travel tapes from the library. John, an excellent golfer and tennis player, especially enjoyed watching these sports on TV. Several days a week, they would have lunch at a restaurant and enjoy an afternoon ride. Evelyn thought she had the days well planned.

Charlie knew the Alzheimer's journey well. He had cared for his own parents, one with AD. Charlie convinced Evelyn that even with the careful plans she was carrying out, she could not provide the much-needed stimulation that John would receive at an adult daycare center. The stimulation that can be experienced in group activities is far superior to that which can be generated in a one-on-one program. Daycare would offer much diversity and a dimension not possible at home: socialization with people experiencing cognitive losses similar to his own.

Charlie was able to help Evelyn see that she was the one resisting daycare. She wasn't ready. John was. He was really ready! Evelyn has always been grateful to Charlie for opening her eyes. He is an example of the important role friends can play on the Alzheimer's journey.

Evelyn visited three adult daycare facilities, notebook in hand. She selected the one that had the most plusses on her chart, chose Tuesday and Thursday to be the daycare days, and chose to provide her own transportation. She followed the advice of the center's social worker and didn't tell John until the Monday night before he was to go.

"Honey, tomorrow we are going to visit a senior center." John didn't react. Later she realized he didn't understand what she was telling him.

Tuesday morning they set off for the daycare center with only a few words of explanation. Evelyn was scared. What if John wouldn't want to stay? How would she handle that? But in addition to fear, she was experiencing a true sense of mourning. More than the early symptoms, more than the accumulation of cognitive losses, more than even the diagnosis, this was the event that spelled it out. She was losing her husband, bit by bit.

Once at the center, Evelyn tucked a piece of notepaper in John's shirt pocket, with the message, "John, I will pick you up at 3:30. I love you." She kissed him good-bye and left quickly. On the fifteen-minute drive home she stopped three times to wipe the tears from her eyes and blow her nose. Once at home, she really cried.

Each day it was easier to take John to daycare. Then, two weeks later, John refused to go. Evelyn asked him, "If I go with you, will you go?" Reluctantly John agreed. Once at daycare, John was met by the official greeter who hugged him, took his coat, and led him to an activity room. Evelyn stood there dumbfounded. John hadn't given a backward glance as he walked in to greet his friends. The social worker took Evelyn, crying once again, into her office. Through the one-way mirror they could watch John. He was obviously enjoying himself.

The social worker was reassuring, saying that if John had acted unhappy or distressed, they would have called her. Often, she said, daycare participants will not admit they are enjoying themselves. About two months later, on a Wednesday (not daycare day), John was fidgety. Evelyn asked, "John, if you had your 'druthers,' what would you like to do?" John's answer surprised and pleased her. "I'd like to go to 'that place.'"

Evelyn assured him they would add another day to his schedule. Eventually John went to daycare five days a week. It became his regular routine. He thoroughly enjoyed his days there. As caring for John became more difficult, Evelyn knew it was daycare that made it possible for her to keep John at home. She has said many times, "I don't know how I would have managed without daycare."

John's life was enriched by his daycare experience. The staff was not focused on John's cognitive losses. Instead they looked for all the ways in which he could participate in the daily activities. They used the skills he still had. He met success every day. He bonded with the other residents. They became buddies, helping one another. John had a life, a purpose, and a routine that brought him great satisfaction.

Every time John brought home one of his woodworking products, the truth of his success was reinforced. He was still there, working hard and producing. He gave an adorable turtle stool to a neighbor's son who was just learning to use the potty. Many people are still using his napkin holders. His Easter basket comes out every year. The watermelon doorstop still gets raves. Of course he needed help with these projects, but his own talents and efforts were used in their successful production.

For those still in doubt about the value of daycare, know that this true story is only one of countless hundreds that can be told. As one experienced social worker declared, "Daycare is one of the very best treatments for someone with Alzheimer's. True, not everyone can benefit, but I suspect that at least 80 percent of those with AD will benefit greatly from this experience."

WHAT TO LOOK FOR IN AN ADULT DAYCARE FACILITY

Physical Appearance

Is the center clean and cheerful? Is there enough room to divide the participants into several groups in order to accommodate a variety of activities and a variety of cognitive skills? Are there comfortable chairs? Is there a place to isolate a sick person? Is there a secured area for outside walking? Is there space for outdoor activities, such as gardening?

Fancy decorations and new furniture may look inviting, but they cannot take the place of a caring, competent staff.

Here are some other questions to ask as you consider daycare options.

Staff

Does the staff include a social worker and an activities director? Is there a physician, nurse, or healthcare professional on staff or on call? What training is given to the volunteers? Are all workers trained in dealing with people with dementia? What is the ratio of staff to participants? Are staff and volunteers warm and friendly to family members and participants? How well can they handle behavioral problems? How long has the center been in operation? What is the turnover rate of the staff?

Activity Program

You should ask for a copy of the activity schedule for the week. We want to make sure there is a variety of activities, for example, cooking, crafts, exercise, current events, reminiscing, gardening, in-house parties. Are the participants divided into cognitive groups so that activities can be geared to individual needs? Is there a trained activity director on campus every day?

Nutrition

Are tasty nutritious meals and snacks provided each day? We should visit at mealtime to see for ourselves. Is the food hot and prepared by a kitchen staff who observes public health rules?

Transportation

Does this center provide transportation to and from the facility? If we plan to provide transportation ourselves, is there any provision for an emergency pickup by the center if you are ill or have car problems?

Cost

What are the basic fees? What is the cost of transportation? Are there additional charges for trips or craft materials? What are the charges for extended hours and late pickups, if we provide transportation? Are there any programs providing financial assistance at this center? Who qualifies for such assistance?

Hours

What are the hours of operation for the center? Are there extended hours—AM and PM? Weekend hours? What are the minimum attendance requirements? What is the policy for absence due to illness or vacation?

Clientele

What is the maximum number of participants permitted at this facility as stated in its license? What are the different types of impairments the center is qualified to serve? Will the client's needs be evaluated? How? How often will the client's needs be reevaluated? Can the facility deal with someone in a wheelchair or someone who is incontinent?

Additional Services

Does the center offer counseling for family members? Will the center administer medications? Are there personal care services such as bathing, hair cutting and styling, help with eating, and toileting? Some centers provide podiatry services, blood pressure screening, and physical therapy programs.

You may not require all the services listed above. You should determine which are the most important for you and your loved one and look for them as you tour each facility.

Evelyn discovered, by accident, that the daycare center John attended provided bathing services for a nominal fee. At the monthly support-group meeting, Evelyn asked for tips to ease the problems she had bathing John. He was well over six feet tall and rather unsteady on his feet. He hadn't started refusing to bathe, but Evelyn knew that day was coming. John was not exactly hindering the process, but he certainly wasn't helping. Evelyn was afraid they would both fall, and then what?!

The social worker interrupted Evelyn's tale of woe. "We give baths here at the center. We tell our residents the bath is doctor's orders. The Jacuzzi-like flow of the water soothes their backs." Evelyn arranged immediately for a twice-weekly bath. The relief was so great, it was as if a lead sinker had been removed from her stomach.

Evelyn knew that John was not always cooperative at daycare. The clothes she picked up at the end of bath day sometimes included damp underwear. On that day he had refused to undress completely before getting into the tub. The staff assured Evelyn that there were no problems, and if there were, they would handle them. They said she need have no concerns.

At that point it seemed a good idea to let the barber and the podiatrist take over two more responsibilities. Evelyn decided it was another way to make life easier.

If you live in a rural area, your choice of daycare may be limited. There may be only one daycare center available. It should be a licensed or certified center that provides appropriate activities and care from a well-trained, happy staff. You should get recommendations from a family currently using the facility. You should feel free to ask questions, sit in on an activity, eat the food, and look at the faces of the staff. Do they smile and act appropriately?

DAYCARE KEEPS NANCY AT HOME

George shares a story that gives the daycare experience an added dimension. He tells us, "Daycare made it possible for my wife, Nancy, to live at home while I continued to work. Nancy was diagnosed with Alzheimer's at sixty-five. We thought it was awfully young. I was sixty-two at the time and not ready to retire. Nancy didn't want me to because she knew how much I enjoyed my work. Also, we knew that Alzheimer's could be an expensive disease. It made good sense for me to continue my earning years as a hedge against future expenses.

"Nancy was able to stay at home alone for a few years. Friends and caring neighbors watched out for her and kept her busy. Then came the time when it really wasn't safe for her to be alone. She could no longer work the television and I was afraid she might turn on the stove. She had never wandered, but that was no guarantee that she might not get it into her head to try to find me or one of her friends. I could tell she was beginning to be afraid of being alone by the way she acted when I got home from work. I knew it wasn't fair to leave her home alone anymore. I was still not ready to retire—what to do?

"I considered several options: a daytime companion or assisted living (there was a beautiful one in town and I had looked at it). Then a friend suggested daycare. After visiting several centers, I found one I really liked. It was the activity program and the friendly, happy-looking staff that really impressed me. They also had extended hours to accommodate working family members.

"The daycare option would allow Nancy to remain at home while enjoying all the benefits daycare would give her. I decided to give it a try. It took Nancy a while to adjust. The social worker kept encouraging me to give her time. By the end of the month Nancy had worked into the routine. She now enjoys the friends she has made and loves the staff.

"I know I will have to expect more changes. I will be ready to retire soon; for now, daycare keeps Nancy in her own home."

Daycare placement has answered the needs of many families caring for a loved one with Alzheimer's. George's story tells of one; Evelyn's of another. Then there is the mother living alone; Mom living with her daughter who works full-time; Dad being cared for by Mother, who is in fragile health herself.

Often, in such situations, if we use daycare, we are postponing the need for a more restrictive environment for our loved one. We are keeping him or her at home for as long as possible. If we are resisting the daycare choice, it may be a good idea to have a talk with ourselves to make sure we are not allowing denial to make the rules.

Chapter Nine

"We Examine Our Attitude toward Alzheimer's"
Caring for the Caregiver—Part II

The rule for overcoming fear is to head right into it.

—Anonymous

In chapter 4, we concentrated on the support network available to the caregiver: family, friends, Alzheimer's Association, support groups, respite providers, etc. Caregiving is too difficult to do alone. To be good caregivers, we need to access the help that is available in our communities, our neighborhoods, our families. We must not think we can do it alone. However, that is often our problem. We mistake asking for help for weakness. If we are not able to maintain our regular daily routine, performing all tasks in grand style, it is admitting defeat. We put our backs to the wall and try even harder. What are we trying to prove? We have another layer of denial to peel away. We need a good look at reality. We must not deny the toll this around-the-clock stressful job can take on our bodies.

WAYS TO DEAL WITH THE CHANGES ALZHEIMER'S BRINGS

In this caregiver chapter we are ready to examine our attitude toward the disease and how it affects our lives. Alzheimer's is the reality. We cannot change that. What we can change are our expectations as we gradually accept the fact that our lives are different. We can control our thoughts and thus control our choice of action. When we accept the fact that Alzheimer's is a part of our lives, we become more able to discover ways to deal with the changes it brings.

As the disease progresses, it becomes necessary to adjust some daily routines in order to make them easier and less time consuming. Using a commercial laundry, occasionally simplifying meal preparation, or utilizing a home cleaning service once a month are ways to lighten housekeeping tasks. At first, we may need encouragement to access that help.

Evelyn found out, at a crucial point in her caregiving, that everything could not be done as usual. She was caring for Grandmother with AD, a teenager, and a six-year-old, all at the same time. Her husband was a great help when he was home, but he often worked late hours. Grandmother had a companion living with her in her apartment. The companion seemed to need as much care as Grandmother. With two households to run and four people with varying needs depending on her, Evelyn was running out of steam. It was a caring family member who convinced her she could not keep up this demanding pace.

After some thought, Evelyn decided that beyond everyone's basic safety, there were only three things that were truly important: clean clothes for everyone; tasty, nutritious meals everyday; and a happy mother. "If Mama ain't happy, ain't nobody happy!" (That old saying is so true.) Everything else was icing on the cake. It was then that Evelyn devised the following list.

THE THREE DO'S

This is a life-saving concept that deserves a separate heading. We should all truly take this advice to heart:

- DO have someone help you.
- DO it differently.
- DO not do it.

These do's can be put into practice over a broad spectrum of household tasks. When she has counseled caregivers, Evelyn has found these do's to be most effectively practiced at holiday time when added duties cause stress that result in what has come to be called the "Holiday Blues Syndrome."

ALLEVIATING THE HOLIDAY BLUES

We could speak about generic holidays, but we have chosen to use Christmas as our focus. Though it is a Christian holiday, many others celebrate the secular aspects of the season. We are all bombarded with holiday reminders on television, radio, and in print media. Stores begin displaying Christmas decorations before Thanksgiving—often right after back-to-school sales. Whether religious or not, we cannot hide from the invasive visual and audio reminders that indeed tell us, "Santa is coming to town."

Let's look at how the holiday season affects caregivers and their families. What we learn here can be applied to almost any other religious holiday, anniversary, or birthday celebration.

Christmas is a beautiful time, rich in tradition and memories: a time of magic for children, a time of good cheer, parties, family celebrations. But what about those of us who are caregivers? This may be a time of great stress. We are already living "the 36-hour day." If we are not careful, we will be headed for the holiday blues, brought on by extra work and more stress. We can do something to alleviate the situation.

Let's look at some of the stress and "bluesmakers."

Commercials Depicting the Ideal

Take, for example, the old Anheuser-Busch commercial. It is the ultimate in picturing the holiday season as perfection. If you remember the commercial, the happy family members are riding in a sleigh over fresh snow to the doorway of a beautifully decorated farmhouse, where they will be greeted by gracious hosts. Everyone is happy. All of the family is together. We can almost smell the pine trees and the roasting turkey. We know the tree is trimmed and perfectly wrapped gifts are beneath.

The commercial shows us the perfection that is far from the reality of our own lives. It adds to our own discontent. We yearn for what can never be.

Additional Tasks

There are cards to send, cookies to make, presents to buy and wrap. We decorate, we go to parties. We become emotionally and physically drained.

Memories of Holidays Past

Our selective memories tell us that all was beautiful. We must keep up the traditions. We remember how our loved one was before the onset of AD. The emotions we have tried to control now threaten to engulf us.

Changes in Routines

Our loved one is adversely affected by changes in routine. The addition of holiday decorations may be confusing and even upsetting. Crowded stores, longer wait times at the checkout counters, and higher noise levels all have a negative affect on our loved ones, and therefore on us caregivers.

Visitors

If we have not told our friends of the severity of the disease, we might feel uncomfortable when they visit.

We want family members to recognize the changes in our loved one and to appreciate how hard we are working. We fear that they are taking us for granted.

That is quite a list of stress and bluesmakers. We recognize an overload of work and emotions. We have some decisions to make. We need to make adjustments to our attitude and actions. This is the perfect place for the three do's:

- DO have someone help you.
- DO it differently.
- DO not do it.

Here are concrete suggestions on how to use the three do's. They are often interchangeable.

Gifts

Shop from a catalog. Find one gift for all, e.g., candles, ornaments, bath products. Give gift certificates. Give gifts to nonprofit health, environmental, or social organizations in the name of the person you are gifting. Send cards instead of gifts to some on your list. Following these suggestions will eliminate tiring and upsetting shopping trips.

Christmas Cooking

Regional and family traditions dictate the importance of various Christmas delicacies: cookies (numerous varieties), fruit cake, stollen, etc. Instead of baking these ourselves, we need to feel free to buy them. We cannot fit one more demanding task into our schedule.

Decorations

Scale back this year. Concentrate on the table centerpiece, the door wreath, and a small tree. We don't have to emulate Martha Stewart. Remember that change of any sort may confuse our loved one.

Cards

We don't need to send cards to anyone we will see during the holiday season. We greet them with a hug, a smile, a warm greeting. Those greetings are better than cards. We can cut our list to include only out-of-town family and good friends. And if the task seems daunting, we must give ourselves permission to omit this ritual completely.

Visits

Encourage family and friends to visit in shifts. Our loved one cannot successfully interact with more than a few visitors at a time. All visits should be short.

Holiday Dinner

If our holiday has, in the past, included unwrapping presents before a big dinner, this year try separating the two events. Have the celebratory meal the day or evening before. Make dishes ahead of time and freeze them. Let family members bring casseroles. Buy a cooked turkey or ham from the local supermarket. Serve buffet-style. Use paper plates, disposable napkins, and plastic utensils. They will be festive looking and will eliminate cleanup chores. Have your dinner at someone else's house: a wonderful "do not do it" idea!

Now we need to ask ourselves what task we dislike, dread, and wish we didn't have to do. Then don't do it, do it differently, or give it to someone else to do. The most important thing is: How do we care for our loved one? First, look at the don'ts:

Don't take him shopping in crowded stores. Avoid confusing situations with:
- Too many people
- Too much noise
- Overactive children

Now, do:
- Spend time with our loved one.
- Sing carols with her.
- Look at pictures of Christmases past.
- Take a drive or walk through the neighborhood, looking at decorations and lights.

Let our loved one help:
- Decorate the tree
- Make cookies
- Set the table

As hard as it may be for us to admit, there will come a time when a favorite holiday or celebration will mean nothing to our loved one. It will be just another day.

Evelyn remembers her attempts to make Christmas a special day for her sister-in-law who was living in a healthcare facility. The first year she made sure Helen participated in the gift exchange and the festive dinner. The next year Helen, with declining health, visited long enough to eat dinner with the family. The third year she spent an hour eating a fancy dessert, but even that was too much for her. When she returned to the health center, she looked at Evelyn and said, "Oh, I am so glad to be home."

Religious holidays, birthdays, and other family get-togethers: No one wants to eliminate these important events in a family's life. But the time comes when we need to do them differently.

We need to be honest. Are we trying to prolong a tradition when it is time to end it?

CHANGING THE FOURTH OF JULY CELEBRATION

At her monthly support-group meeting, Andrea told the following story:

"Our annual Fourth of July celebration has always been held at Mom and Dad's house. They have the big backyard where we have our picnic with corn on the cob, crab cakes, hamburgers and hot dogs on the grill, watermelon, and Mom's scrumptious coconut cake. Then there are the games for everyone, young and old: volleyball, horseshoes, and one-on-one basketball. Dad always pulls out the croquet set. We tease him, telling him it's a lady's game. We know he loves to play it because he can always beat us. We tease him about that too. Now that Dad has Alzheimer's disease, Mom works very hard taking care of him. She gets really tired. And Dad has failed so much. We don't know what to do. How can we give up this tradition that means so much to all of us? We grew up on it and now our kids look forward to it as much as we do."

Evelyn suggested this was a perfect place for the three do's. This year, because Dad still enjoys being with his family, the Fourth of July celebration could take place successfully with the first do, "Have someone help you do it," and a little of the second do, "Do it differently." The family members make a list of all the jobs that need to be done to create the treasured celebration, from the setting up to the cleaning up. Everyone gets a job, even the grandchildren. Mom's only job will be to make her scrumptious coconut cake while a family member takes Dad for a ride.

This year the "Do it differently part" refers to a shortened party. Plan to end festivities earlier than usual. Prolonged noise, even happy noise, and continuing activity are wearing and sometimes overstimulating, especially for a person with AD. Next year, the visits can be staggered so Dad only has one of his children's families at a time. This will lower the confusion and fatigue levels. The picnic may just be watermelon and iced tea, and a game of croquet, of course.

It is easy to see that the next do, "Don't do it," is inevitable. When Mom can no longer host the party, she must agree to the third do. The celebration will have to take a different form at one of the children's homes. It won't be the same, but we are adapting to change.

One more word about the three do's before we move on. Whenever we caregivers feel totally worn out, we need to ask ourselves, "Is there some task we could give up, do differently, or give to someone else to do?"

ATTITUDE ADJUSTMENT

As informed caregivers we realize our loved one has a progressive disease. He is as good now as he will ever be. He cannot change. We are the ones who must do the changing.

In an old Peanuts comic strip, Charlie Brown spent the week with a dark cloud over his head. He kept grumbling that no one liked him. He was miserable. At the end of the week, Lucy appeared in the strip with her five-cent advice: "Charlie Brown, lift up your head, smile; it will make you feel better." Charlie replied, "I don't want to feel better."

It was a simple weekly comic strip that packed a whale of a message. Lucy was right. If we stand up and smile, we do feel better. (Try it right now. We guarantee it will make you feel better.) Charlie Brown teaches us an equally important lesson. We have to want to feel better. It's our decision. We cannot change the disease. But we can adjust our attitude.

We need to be realistic about what our loved one can and cannot do. We should not underestimate her cognitive losses. At the same time we must not lose sight of what she can do. This will have a positive effect on our attitude.

At the grocery store, our loved one can help put the items from the basket onto the conveyor belt. At home he can carry small bundles into the kitchen. He can take the items out of the bags and put them on the table as the caregiver puts them in the cupboards. Will he make mistakes? Probably. Will it take longer than if we do it alone? Of course. Will he feel good about having had a job to do? Yes!! That is all the reason we need to include him in any activity in which he can participate.

There are many enjoyable activities we can do with our loved one: short walks in the neighborhood, rides in the country, listening to favorite music, watching videos (the library has many to choose from), looking at old photo albums. We can bake together. She may only stir the batter a little, cut out one or two cookies, or sprinkle the sugar on top. But she knows she has helped. She hasn't been pushed aside. It may get messy in the kitchen. The task will take longer. The reward? Our loved one will feel loved. And we will have connected with her in a way that will benefit us both.

Susie tells us of the time she and her dad with AD colored Easter eggs together. "We each wore those coverup aprons, but I made sure everything else we had on was washable. I wasn't sure Dad would take to the task. He had never done anything like that when he was well. But you know, he got such a big kick out of seeing those eggs turn different colors. He wasn't as interested in the decals. He just wanted to dip the eggs and watch them turn colors. I was so glad I decided to let him help. It makes me feel so good to see him smile."

Fred shared the "poker chip sorting tale." Fred kept his poker chips in the bottom drawer of his desk. When his children were young they loved to pull open that drawer and play with the chips. They made up all sorts of games that kept them busy for hours. One day Fred was caring for his mother with AD. He wanted to engage her in an activity that she might enjoy. Fred tells us, "I thought of my kids and the poker chips. It was worth a try. Maybe Mom and I could play with them. We sat at the dining room table. First we separated them into colors. Then we put them in piles until they fell over. We made rows of alternating colors. Then we went back to sorting them. I actually had fun. I know Mom did. We laughed a lot; more than we had in ages. That day taught me that Mom and I could still do things together and have fun."

Attitude adjustment can begin when we focus on the positives in our lives. When we can make our loved ones laugh and enjoy an activity, we have given them a gift that we can share. Our loved ones will not remember the happy event but they will remember the emotion. That happy feeling stays with them.

Our attitude adjustment begins with changing the way we look at our loved ones' lives. We try to focus on what they can do, not on what they cannot do. Now it's time to look at the caregivers' lives. What can we do to bring beauty, joy, and laughter into our own lives? We could easily get caught up in all the demanding details and claim we have no time for that nonsense.

TAKING CARE OF THE CAREGIVER

Here is another layer of the denial onion. Because the job is so demanding, we cannot overlook our own emotional, spiritual, and physical needs. We cannot be the best caregivers unless we take care of ourselves.

Evelyn drove her husband to daycare over the same route each day. It was more than a month before she noticed "the tree." It was a twelve-foot weeping cherry tree in full bloom, so beautiful that she wanted to stop and feast her eyes on the magnificent sight. She wondered why she had not noticed it before. How could she have missed such beauty? Now each day she looked forward to seeing the cherry tree. She began calling it her "thank-you-God" tree. It was beautiful even after the blooms had faded and fallen. She had the visual treat four times a day.

That was the beginning of Evelyn's looking for the beauty that surrounded her. By November she was used to looking for beauty in the ordinary and had no trouble appreciating the bare oak and elm branches silhouetted against the gray sky. What once might have been a dreary sight was now something beautiful to lift her spirits.

We invite you, the tired caregiver, to look for the beauty in your life. It may be in the music you love or the laughter of your grandchild. It may be the flowering fruit tree outside your window, the plants on your windowsill, the weeping willow trees swaying in the breeze, the smell of garlic in bubbling tomato sauce. Just look, smell, feel, hear; you will find beauty in the small moments of your life. Eating a piece of chocolate is a known mood enhancer!

Now we invite you to plan some things that are pleasant to look forward to. These need not be extraordinary events. They can be the ordinary elements in your life, but now you are going to consciously look forward to them with pleasure. Some events may need actual planning; others need just a little tweaking to make them special.

Evelyn found herself looking forward to reading that special book from the library (tip: if it isn't on the shelf, put the book you'd really like to read on hold), an afternoon with a friend, or a bubble bath with bubbles up to her chin. We can look forward to our favorite TV show; Sunday afternoon sports; renting a funny movie. Those of us who are cooks can plan a different meal with new recipes. The gardener can pore over plant and seed catalogs and plan the spring/summer garden.

We are taking the ordinary and making it special, because we want it to be special. Oh, what power our own thoughts can have!

We want to plan treats for our loved one, to recapture and remember past joys as we look together at pictures from the happy times in our past—vacations, school days, honeymoon. Our loved one can remember the distant past but not yesterday. Play the music that once inspired your loved one to dance. Sing the songs that were so popular in his or her youth. The joy you bring into your loved one's life will be doubled in your own.

Because the disease is never ending, we need to be kind to ourselves:

- We need to eat healthy meals, and we need to exercise. Exercise is a great stress reducer. Take a walk around the block and look for beauty. Walk in the mall when it's icy or during hot summer days.
- We must schedule regular visits to the doctor.
- Take one day at a time. Don't borrow tomorrow. When the days are particularly difficult, take the day one hour at a time.
- Have someone to talk with, such as a telephone buddy.
- Keep a journal. We don't have to write every day, but do try to write at the end of a difficult day. We need not worry about grammar, punctuation, or spelling. No one else will see what we write. We need a place to freely express our frustrations, anger, and fear. *And this is important*: end every entry with at least three things we are thankful for, even if one of them is that we are thankful the day is over.

- Practice positive "self-talk." We need to tell ourselves, aloud, several times a day: "I am doing a good job!" We need to say it even when we make a mistake; we cannot be perfect.
- Treat ourselves to a new hairdo, a golf game.
- We should laugh often and laugh with our loved one with Alzheimer's.
- Access respite, by using the help of friends, family, and daycare.

When we take care of ourselves, we are not being selfish.

Reach out to people; maintain friendships. We must not get caught in the cul-de-sac of Alzheimer's disease. We must keep walking toward the avenue bathed in sunlight.

It is all right to cry, with Evelyn's light-hearted caveat: set the timer; stop when the bell rings.

In the words of Shakespeare:

> Give sorrow words,
> Grief that does not speak
> Knits up the human heart
> And bids it break.

As we take charge and practice some (or all) of these sound pieces of advice, the knowledge will come to us: we are making a positive difference in our own life and in the life of our loved one. The more we practice love of self, the more love we have to give.

As we adjust our attitude to gain a proper perspective, we find ourselves able to smile and laugh. This produces the environment that fosters patience.

Patience: we can never have too much of it!

Chapter Ten

"I Only Promised because She Made Me"
The Long-term Care Decision

**The arms of love encompass you with your present, your
past, your future; the arms of love gather you together.**

—Antoine de St-Exupéry

One of the more difficult things we have to do in life is face
unpleasant realities. When that reality involves the failing health of
a loved one and necessitates a change as drastic as placement in a long-term
care facility, denial often takes over. It protects us from ideas, concepts, and
especially facts that we are not ready to handle. But when our loved one's
capacity for self-direction and self-care diminishes drastically due to AD,
and, as caregivers we are no longer able to meet his or her needs, we must
work through our denial and take action.

For everything there is a season. There is a time for everything, and
nothing lasts forever (except love!). We caregivers must take a long, honest
look at our own lives and the lives of our failing loved one. In the progression of Alzheimer's disease, there is a strong likelihood that some form of
supportive-care placement will be necessary. This is the difficult reality to
face. We see the albatross (denial) playing a big part in our avoidance of
making this decision. Sometimes our reluctance can even be at the expense
of our own health and the well-being of our loved one.

There are thoughts and observations that should alert us to the fact
that we need to examine Mom's or Dad's living situation thoroughly and
talk things over with other family members:

- "Mom has lived in her home for more than forty years and doesn't ever want to leave it. However, sometimes she seems so isolated and overwhelmed."
- "Dad moved to an apartment many years ago after losing Mom. He has adjusted and seems to be happy there. But is he able to manage his own care?"

We have many and varied reasons for reluctance and procrastination. One reason is that our whole culture is in denial about aging; or at least any visible form of it. There is no cure for our own mortality. It is difficult to accept the fact that we are born, we live, we grow old (if we're lucky!), and we die. In our Western culture, youth and the "movers and shakers" get the attention. Ergo, it truly does take a major effort to break through the collective social as well as personal denial.

We authors believe that no one should try to shoulder Alzheimer's caregiving responsibilities alone. Even with the best of intentions—being independent, "not burdening anyone"—it is not a good idea. That is why we urge family members of loved ones with AD to get involved in a support group as early as possible in the caregiving process. Placement of a loved one is a difficult reality to face; the shared information, experience, and support of a group of other caregivers will prove invaluable. It is very comforting and helps us resolve our feelings of guilt. We caregivers are often afflicted with some form of "primordial guilt" that seems to be built into our psyches. We believe we should be able to meet all the needs of our loved one—meet any challenge, face any adversity. If we do not live up to our own expectations, we feel we have failed. There is always someone we know who is managing everything successfully. We know that some other societies manage to care for their elderly at home—and our guilt multiplies.

We might have built up routines with our loved ones that seem to be meeting their needs. We visit daily, shop for them, and even provide them with in-home support services. Or, we might be caring for them in our home or in theirs. We might not yet be willing to even consider the fact that our loved ones could receive more comprehensive care and have their needs better met in a residential care center.

Summed up, our reasons for procrastination include feelings of guilt and denial of the mortality of our loved one, as well as our own mortality. We must move through this part of our journey and enter the action phase.

IS IT TIME?

Regardless of the degree to which these issues remain in play, or how mercurial our thoughts, eventually we must face the big question: *Is it time?*

We can use as guidelines the activities of daily living (often referred to as ADLs) and the functions of daily living to make an assessment of our loved one's basic abilities.

The ADLs include:
- Dressing
- Hygiene (bathing, etc.)
- Feeding
- Toileting (bladder and bowel control)
- Mobility (The ability to get in and out of a bed or chair. If in a wheelchair, the ability to transfer to and from bed or chair.)

The basic functions of daily living include:
- Shopping
- Cooking
- Using the telephone
- Light housekeeping
- Administering medications
- Keeping track of simple finances
- Arranging for necessary transportation

If our loved one continues to live alone, he or she should be able to perform the ADLs with little or no help. As the disease progresses, our loved one will lose the ability, in an unpredictable pattern, to perform basic functions. It is usually easy to determine when our loved one needs help with shopping, housekeeping, transportation, managing finances. We are not always as aware that our loved one is not able to prepare proper meals or self-administer medications. If we ask Mother what she had for dinner, she can recite an appealing menu. But can we believe her? Remember, she is keeping her social graces and recalls appropriate answers to many questions.

Back to the big question: Is it time? How do we know when it would be in our loved one's best interest to be moved to a more supportive environment?

Here are the major indicators that "it is time" when our loved one lives alone:

- Inability to perform the AD's
- Inability to self-administer daily medications and/or insulin injections
- Frequent falls
- Wandering
- Possibility of leaving stove unattended
- Needing many assistive devices, e.g., cane, walker, emergency alert system—and forgetting to use them

The following are major indicators when our loved one lives with family members:

- Caregiver suffers from significant health problems.
- Caregiver becomes too physically and/or emotionally exhausted to give proper care.
- Caregiver works all day, leaving loved one alone when problems, such as wandering or leaving the stove unattended, may arise.
- While caregiver is at work, loved one is bored, sleeps a lot, and is awake much of the night.
- Caregiver takes so much time off from work to care for loved one's needs that his or her job is in jeopardy.
- Loved one needs more care than working caregiver can give.
- Caregiver cannot afford to stop working.

After researching, soul searching, and getting the doctor's opinion, we come to the conclusion that our loved one—Mom, Dad, spouse, or another close relative—has reached the point where some form of placement is necessary. We continue to hesitate. A primary reason for delay—that we haven't wanted to face as yet—is the promise we made to ourselves: "I will never place my loved one in a nursing home," or the promise we made to our loved one, at their insistence: "I will always take care of you. You will never have to live in a nursing home." If this promise has already been made, whether to yourself or to your loved one, there are creative and constructive ways to manage its fallout. If you are lucky and have not yet made this promise, do not do it! Never make a promise you may not be able to keep. These kinds of promises, even when made in good faith, can have negative consequences.

> **TIP:** *For those who find themselves trapped in this situation, we have a suggestion. We need to reassure ourselves and our loved one that we have given them the very best care at home for as long as possible. Now, we will continue to be the primary caregiver in a new setting. "I promised to do my best and that is what I have done and will continue to do." This approach can free the caregiver to make a promise with a caveat. Caregivers breaking down physically or emotionally does not help matters. Again, our mantra:* I can't take care of my loved one unless I take care of myself.

It is natural for new caregivers, just starting out on the Alzheimer's journey with a loved one, to become anxious when reading or hearing anything concerning nursing homes and placement issues. The fear we have for our loved one includes our fear for our own future—however far off it may seem. After all, we wouldn't want anyone "putting us away"!

We can hear words of denial and protest:

"What do you mean, send my father to a nursing home?"

"I am never going to put my wife away!"

"I have no intention of letting anyone else take care of my mother—that's my job!"

"No one knows my husband the way I do or can provide for his needs the way I can."

What are we really hearing when we listen to the above kinds of reasoning? We hear the sound of fear. Old tapes from previous generations are playing in our heads. Most of our fears and worries are based on things we have heard and seen in the past, especially the things we heard while growing up. It is the "echo" of fear. Most of those tales and legends were based on another time. After all, the folks we heard them from had heard them from *their* previous generation. Old myths and mores die hard. We also fear people judging us as weak if we can not meet our loved one's needs. And hidden in our hearts is fear for our own future. Fear magnifies everything in a false and even grotesque way, as we imagine ourselves losing our own independence someday. No doubt, that is one of the things we most dread as we go through life. We don't want anyone telling us what to do.

> **TIP:** *Never use the phrase* put away. *This phrase is an unfortunate part of the vocabulary of previous generations and previous centuries. It clearly indicates how the power of the spoken word can cause so much pain and strong feelings of rejection. We live in a rapidly changing world. The poor houses, work farms, and institutions where people were "put away" were part of the early twentieth century and no longer exist. We do not "put people away." When it is deemed necessary, responsible family members "place" their loved ones in cheerful, well-staffed nursing centers where their needs can be better met.*

Society in general does not keep up with the changing times. Things change and later, sometimes much later, society catches up with those changes intellectually and emotionally. We are a highly adaptive species, but any kind of change frightens us, even if it is good change, known as "progress." There has been much progress in the long-term care industry. Perhaps visiting a long-term care facility might change some of those old beliefs.

Residential healthcare facilities vary in price, number of occupants, and amount of care and support they provide. We will mention all of them, but only go into detail on the options that would be appropriate for our loved ones with AD. While the reader is experiencing virtual tours and stories of actual placements, it will become clear that much thought will be involved in the placement decision. No matter what level of care is needed for our loved one, the whole process from start to finish requires courage and effort on everyone's part.

Previous chapters have dealt with family meetings and how important they are. By now some of our family members should have had a meeting in person or in a conference call to discuss the needs of our loved one with dementia. Placement is at the top of the list of denial issues involving Alzheimer's disease; families usually make the placement decision only after every other option has been ruled out. Therefore, we will proceed with care as we examine our choices. If our loved one is in the hospital as the option is being considered, it is important to include the social worker or nurse case manager in the decision making. Their expertise will make the process much easier. Whether at home or in the hospital, the situation can be examined from all angles, with everyone who is willing, having input.

Once our family has agreed that their loved one needs the level of care that cannot be achieved in the home setting, we should discuss all possible solutions, weighing the pros and cons before making the choice between one of the several forms of placement. We can then proceed with information gathering while keeping our attitude as positive as possible.

By now the people involved in this decision are trying to get on the same page. These meetings and discussions must necessarily exclude our loved one. We want to include him or her as much as possible, but during the fact-finding phase of placement and during visits to various facilities, it is not a good idea. It can be a source of worry and anxiety for someone who is confused. Later, appropriate decisions can be presented, e.g., what pictures and knickknacks to bring along, where to place belongings, etc. (Occasionally a loved one might have already chosen a particular facility while he or she is still competent. There is such a story later in this chapter.)

We want to look for a facility that is committed to providing care for persons with dementia. It is imperative that the home we choose has a philosophy that addresses our loved one's needs. We might be faced with deciding whether we prefer our loved one to be in a homogeneous or integrated setting, i.e., only with others with dementia or with people with different problems related to aging. There are benefits to both. We should discuss this with the staff at the various facilities we visit and make an informed decision. It is very important to find out whether the facility can provide care for our loved one throughout the progression of the disease. Once in a residential setting, it is better not to move those who have settled in and become accustomed to the surroundings and caregivers. But if it can't be avoided, we should not lose heart over it.

There are several types of facilities that provide care for our loved ones with dementia, from the least restrictive to the most supportive.

MULTIPLE AND DIVERSE RESIDENTIAL HEALTHCARE SETTINGS

Board and Care/Adult Boarding Homes/ Adult Foster Homes or Group Homes

Sometimes regulated by the state, boarding or foster homes are important alternatives for those who need some assistance but who are not totally dependent. They are less expensive than the other options because they are private homes that have been transformed to provide for group care. The rooms may be private or semiprivate. Meals are provided, along with various amounts of care assistance and some structured activities. At licensed, smaller group homes, care tends to be more personalized. They often provide a warm, supportive environment for our loved one. It is a matter of finding the right match. Be sure to carefully check the staffing. Is there a nurse on the premises or on call? Visit the kitchen; talk to those who prepare the food; check out the menu.

If a guest cannot pay privately, Medicaid waivers might cover this type of housing. The local Alzheimer's Association office, the department on aging, or the department of social services should have information on those homes. Ask for the facility Web site where more specific information can be found.

Assisted Living Facilities

Regulated by the state, these facilities are for those who need some form of assistance with their activities of daily living (ADLs)—eating, bathing, dressing, toileting, mobility. Some of the large chains around the country are quite appealing, in providing both a good program and a pleasant environment. They are often of new construction and can be lovely to look at both inside and out. They can also be expensive. We are not going to discuss costs because they vary from state to state and they change rapidly. When people have the resources to pay the rates for assisted living facilities, it is important that they think ahead to when they may need a higher level of care. That is even more expensive.

Assisted living facilities can be appropriate for persons in the early to middle stages of Alzheimer's. Some facilities even allow families to privately fund "sitters," thereby keeping the loved one in one place throughout the disease process. Other facilities may not be able to keep people beyond a certain level of care, requiring them to move. It is very important to establish up front if the facility will be able to keep our loved one throughout the course of the illness.

It is also important, when choosing an assisted living or a long-term care facility, that families do as much research as possible. The ratio of staff to residents is critical. More than six patients per caregiver likely is stretching the caregiver to the max. Check with the local department on aging or the state attorney general's office as to whether there have been any complaints against the chosen facility. Again, the Alzheimer's Association, the department on aging, or the department of social services can provide lists of such homes. Some of them have Medicaid waiver beds, usually with long waiting lists.

When Evelyn took charge of her sister-in-law's care, Helen was living independently in a neighboring state, a three-hour journey away. Helen was in the early stages of Alzheimer's disease and knew she needed different living arrangements. She chose an apartment in a beautifully appointed assisted living facility. Evelyn's first job was to plan and oversee her move. Helen was very happy in her new home, making friends and participating in many social programs. Evelyn was working part-time and thus able to spend two long weekends a month with Helen, taking care of her personal and financial affairs. John, also in the early stages of AD, accompanied Evelyn on each trip. He was happy spending time with his sister.

Helen was living in what was considered to be the finest assisted living facility in her state. However, it was early in the development of appropriate care for dementia residents—the early 1990s. The facility did not have a locked unit. When Helen started to wander, sometimes miles from the facility, it was time to consider a different placement. (After Helen's move, her assisted living facility created a locked unit. Evelyn saw other positive advances in dementia care facilities over the years.)

Evelyn decided to move Helen to a nursing facility with an excellent Alzheimer's unit, located less than ten minutes from her home. Evelyn agonized over the way she would tell Helen about the move. Not only would Helen be moving from a home she had known for two years, but also she would be moving away from friends and a city she had known for forty years. Evelyn practiced breaking the news to Helen in front of a mirror with a written script. Helen was still in the early stages of the disease and would have a fair understanding of what was happening. Evelyn wanted to put the best spin on the coming move.

Once again, as with Grandmother's move, Evelyn need not have worried. Helen was delighted to know that she would now be close to her brother and sister-in-law. She would be with them more often than twice a month. It was as if she were moving closer to her security base. She had only one worry.

"Evelyn," she asked, "do you think they will like me?"

For the next six years, Helen lived in a healthcare facility that not only "liked her," but also provided her with loving care, mental and social stimulation, and friends with whom she formed strong bonds.

TIP: *We must not fear the nursing home choice. We still are the main caregivers. We can oversee all that happens to our loved one. When we form a working relationship with the staff at the nursing center, we create a team stronger than the individual components. Evelyn still exchanges Christmas cards with the nurses who cared for Helen.*

Continuing Care Communities/Retirement Communities/ Life Care Facilities

Regulated by the state, these communities provide the most comprehensive setting, which includes independent living, assisted living, and a skilled nursing facility all on one campus. All of the residents' care needs can be met at the different levels. Overall, they can be very suitable for those who can afford them. People who own their homes outright and are able to obtain a good price for them are best suited financially. However, they will also need substantial pension and social security checks, as these communities increase their monthly fees regularly. Once accepted financially and medically, a person or a couple will be in a community that will continue providing care even if the money runs out and the resident must rely on Medicaid/Medicare. That's good news. Some of these communities return funds invested in the condo/apartment to the resident's estate upon death, others do not.

These communities are made up of different living levels, depending on the level of support needed. Residents usually enter at the completely independent level. They live in a condo/apartment (sometimes called a patio home or a cottage), and they can have their own car. The main meal is included; laundry and housework is done weekly or biweekly; and there are other amenities. There is an emergency response system—typically, a pendant with an emergency button, which can be pushed if someone falls or feels faint. There is also an emergency pull cord in the bathroom and a bedside emergency response system. Many residents feel cozy and safe.

It is suggested that people move when they are still well and can make the decision for themselves, so they can meet people, form bonds, and feel comfortable and at home. But many refuse to even consider these options until the last possible minute, when catastrophe is ready to strike. Another one of those bad ideas! If we can afford to enter a retirement community when we are still well and our spouse is in the early stages of dementia, it is better to go sooner rather than later. Some might accept a couple if one person has dementia and the other is capable of handling the situation, until placement in the assisted living or nursing unit becomes necessary. Or sometimes the couple enters the community with one in an apartment and the other going directly into assisted living or the nursing unit. If they have two units, then two costs are incurred. Some places do not accept couples unless both are competent and can care for themselves.

Another possible configuration is a single person over sixty-two (the usual age for acceptance) who has an elderly parent with dementia. This arrangement can work well until the care needs of the parent become overwhelming. Then the parent may be moved into either the assisted living or nursing care unit. These are part of the same community and on the same campus.

It is important to remember that these communities are expensive and are not appropriate for everyone. They are listed in the telephone book, at the local Alzheimer's Association, and at the state or county department of aging. In addition to touring the independent units, we need to look closely at the assisted living section and nursing facility. Again, we are looking for an adequate patient-aide ratio and stimulating activity programs. At some of the continuing care communities, more money and effort go into the independent living program than into the nursing care facility, where the need is greater. For this reason alone, we need to be careful shoppers.

Long-term Care Facilities/Nursing Homes/ Skilled Nursing Facilities/Healthcare Centers

Whether state and/or federally regulated, these facilities are focused on providing a medically supportive environment. For those who are in need of what they provide, they are the best and sometimes the only choice. But they are expensive and Medicare contributes little, if anything to the cost. Even then, it pays only for a short time—a matter of weeks—when someone is receiving care for a condition that can be improved, e.g., physical therapy for a hip fracture, wound care, or injections. These are examples of conditions that meet Medicare requirements for a "skilled level of care."

Throughout our tour, we want to be aware of the attitude of the staff and the expressions on their faces. When we enter the facility, are we greeted with a smile? Are staff members seen interacting in a positive way with the residents? Are they responsive to questions when asked? Do they have an air of competence and confidence about them? Do they seem friendly? If we get a sense that staff members are just marking time until their shift ends, or they look bored, annoyed, or put-upon, that's not a good sign.

Nursing facilities can be beautiful to look at and many are highly desirable for placement of our loved ones; but frankly, many are not. If there is no bad odor when entering the home, that is a good omen. If we are bowled over by the nasty aroma, we should leave immediately. No explanation is necessary. It is nonnegotiable. They will get the message and maybe they will do better next time. There is no excuse for it! Most facilities do not schedule tours when rooms are being cleaned and patients bathed and changed. Also, be aware of heavy cover-up sprays—not a good sign, either.

We should also take note of whether the residents are sitting around, slumped in wheelchairs with blank facial expressions. Obviously residents have the right to be out in the halls and not stuck in their rooms all day, but we should never walk in the front door of a facility and be greeted with that scene.

We should allow luck to play only as small a part as possible in choosing a long-term care facility for our loved one. We can do that by digging in and doing extensive research on the appropriateness of the facilities we visit. Some things will be left to chance, as we cannot handpick the caregivers for our loved one.

If the decision for placement is made, we must become aware of the many issues to come.

> **TIP:** *Some of the most important people who care for our loved ones in any institutional setting are the CNAs—Certified Nursing Assistants. The approach, attitude, and demeanor of these caregivers are critical. If they are basically pleasant persons who reflect generosity of spirit, this will flow into their job of working with the frail elderly. This is very important. If the opposite is true, it may not be a good environment for our loved one. Obviously the professional caregiver will change with shifts, vacations, and the comings and goings of new employees. It is important that we monitor the actions of these caregivers. The night shift is difficult to check. One might make it a priority to get to the nursing home early in the morning, at least occasionally, before the shift changes; or stay at night until the shift changes to meet the staff. We must be careful, always, to treat all shifts equally if we choose to write notes of appreciation or give boxes of candy or fruit baskets at holiday times. If our means won't permit gifting, a card with a written note of thanks will be much appreciated.*

The nurses in charge at each shift are very important. They oversee everyone on the floor, dispense medications, and keep the unit running smoothly. We must make sure to remember them when we are generously sprinkling our gratitude around. If a problem occurs with a staff member, it should be discussed promptly with that staff member.

If our general rapport is good with everyone in the facility, problems often can be smoothed out easily. Sometimes the problem is a misperception or misunderstanding. The key is to deal with a problem immediately. This keeps it from continuing or becoming magnified. If this avenue does not rectify the situation, we can approach the head of the unit. We want to try to avoid having any of the aides or nurses singled out or reprimanded. If that becomes necessary, however, we should not shrink from it. As a last resort, we can put complaints in writing or contact the ombudsman.

QUESTIONS TO ASK WHEN VISITING A NURSING FACILITY

Here are a few direct questions to ask when visiting a nursing facility:

- How does this facility address the unique needs of people with dementia?
- What is the ratio of aides to residents?
- How often does the staff meet with families for updates?
- What role does the family have in problem solving?
- Are there support groups and is there a family council?
- How are issues and concerns resolved?
- How open are staff members to special requests made by family members for their loved ones? (For example, Mom needs to have someone turn on the TV every afternoon so she can watch *Oprah*.)
- Is there an activity director?

In some states, nursing homes are required to keep a book that describes the yearly state assessment. It should be readily available for all to read.

Before placement in any facility, it is important for residents to have durable powers of attorney set up—both medical and financial. Information about patients' rights and the Nursing Home Ombudsman Program should be made available to the "responsible party" for each resident. (This program handles unresolved problems a customer may have with any given facility.)

Again, nursing homes are expensive. People who have been wise enough to purchase long-term care insurance will have some relief, but even it may not cover everything for the duration of the stay. Some private facilities do not have Medicaid beds. But a certain number of Medicaid waiver beds are licensed in most facilities (check with your local department of social services). They are sometimes difficult to find in the facility of our choice and our loved one may be placed on a waiting list. Going directly to a nursing center from the hospital can sometimes alleviate this problem. Due to the need for hospitals to discharge patients quickly and efficiently, nursing homes usually accept hospital patients before prospective residents in the community, especially when beds are at a premium. But even here, many nursing homes will prefer private pay residents to those on public assistance.

The Alzheimer's Association, the hospital, the department on aging, or the department of social services can provide lists of nursing facilities.

> **TIP:** *If we can earmark (save) enough money to cover three to six months of private pay, our loved one can usually be accepted into the nursing home of our choice. Even when we need to apply for the government assistance program, our loved one can stay in the facility.*

Ellen and Evelyn have both had their own experiences with placing loved ones in nursing facilities.

Ellen's mother, Mary Alice, was in her late seventies when she said she might someday like to go to a nursing home around the corner from where she was living. Although two of her friends already lived there, she made it clear that she wasn't quite ready yet. "Maybe someday in the distant future." Ellen remembered that discussion. It predicted the possibility of her mother being able to make some of the decisions.

For the next two years Ellen used her medical social work skills to put support systems in place for her mother. Mary Alice had homemaker services three days a week, a walker, a bedside commode, and an emergency response pendant to wear around her neck.

As most people do, Mary Alice struggled to remain independent, sending the companion home when she felt she didn't need her. One time when Ellen arrived for a visit, she got off the elevator to be greeted by Mary Alice standing in the hallway in her slip. Ellen said, "Oh, Mother, you must be cold, you only have your slip on. Quick, let's get into your apartment [which was only a short distance] and get you in a robe." As she put on the robe, Mary Alice said, "I guess that was an odd thing to do, wasn't it—to go out with only my slip on?"

Ellen brushed it off lightly, but it was definitely out of character and just one more indicator of the encroaching dementia. It had attacked her mother's capacity for self-awareness, which is critical to retaining one's "alert and oriented" status. That incident alone might have had little meaning. But Ellen knew that, as a part of the whole picture, it was significant and was just another sign that the time was coming. They went to see the nursing home, and while touring the facility, Mary Alice said, "I hope I don't give you a hard time, Ellen." Even at her level of confusion, she was still high on the "thoughtful" scale. On the way home, she said, "It's not something I really want to do, but if you want me to and feel that it is best, I will go. I do, after all, have two friends who already live there."

That was a moment of clarity, a moment when Ellen's mother had insight and intention. Ellen remembered those words, knowing they were being said in a moment when Mary Alice knew what she was saying. Soon thereafter, when the going got tough, Ellen reminded her of her words. Because she was quite forgetful, Mary Alice did not remember saying those things but graciously acknowledged that she knew Ellen wouldn't say so unless she had.

The final straw came when the woman living next door to Mary Alice told Ellen that the police had come the night before. Mary Alice had fallen and was unable to get up. She had tapped on the wall until the neighbor called for help. The police actually had to break into her apartment to help her. Mary Alice had asked that Ellen not be told, saying she didn't want to worry her. But Ellen believed the more pressing reason to be that her mother knew "it was time."

The move to the nursing home actually went rather smoothly. All of the difficulties had been discussed at length and dealt with before moving day.

During the first few months that Mary Alice was a resident of the nursing facility, she had a lovely room on the first floor. She could walk around and see everything, including going out on the patio and sitting on a bench under her favorite tree. One day, however, she was overcome by "wanderlust." Ellen was informed that her mother had been found strolling around the Rotunda shopping center across the street from the nursing home. She was having a great time, window shopping and exploring.

Mary Alice's behavior did not fit the nursing home's requirements. She was moved to the second floor where she received a security bracelet. Attempting to get on the elevator would set off an alarm at the nurses' station. On a happy note, she never tried. She seemed content to stay on her floor.

TIP: *We should try to remember any clear statements made by our loved ones in moments when their generosity of spirit trumps their fear. These moments do exist, but they often go unnoticed during stressful times. We should remember them and if the appropriate moment arises,* use them as gentle nudges or reminders. We all have the ability to rise above our "selves." Most people would like to appear brave in the face of adversity. We do not want to impose troubles on others, especially our family and friends. Gentle discussions of "how brave our loved one is or how brave we know he or she will be" can gently nudge him or her out of a self-indulgent pity party and into a more insightful generosity of spirit.

IMPORTANCE OF ADVANCE PLANNING

Evelyn's experience with her husband's nursing home placement underscores the importance of advance planning. Caring for John was becoming more difficult. Just getting him to bed each night took every bit of patience Evelyn could muster. She finally hired the woman who gave him baths at daycare to help her with the wearing task. In addition, John resisted taking needed medication. His frustrations often resulted in anger directed at Evelyn. Friends and family members suggested that it might be time to consider nursing home placement.

Evelyn was not ready for this move, but she took the advice she always gave to her support-group members: look ahead and be prepared for the changes that occur in the course of the disease. After visiting several nursing centers, Evelyn chose the one that ran John's daycare. He was evaluated and deemed appropriate for admission. Evelyn could make the move when she was ready.

It is often unexpected events that dictate needed action. Several weeks later, John suffered a stroke and seizure. He was taken to the hospital and four days later entered the chosen nursing facility. Evelyn was grateful that she had been prepared. She knew the wisdom of being ready for unexpected turns of events, because the future is so uncertain.

If we are having difficulty convincing our loved one of the wisdom of the move to a care facility, a sometimes forgotten ally to call on for support is the doctor. Physicians can help soften the blow if their relationships are good with our loved ones. They can appear to be more objective than family members. Often people will listen to a doctor when they resent being "told what to do" by adult children or other close family members.

This idea is certainly worth a try. Depending on where our loved one is on the scale of dementia, this may or may not be a problem. (Review the "rearrange reality" technique in chapter 6.)

TWENTY-FOUR-HOUR PROFESSIONAL CARE AT HOME

Another option is to keep our loved one in the home setting by providing appropriate staff to meet his or her care needs there. This is the least recommended choice for persons in the middle and late stages of AD. From a practical standpoint, it is very expensive to have round-the-clock nursing care in the home for what might be many years. When our loved one's financial resources are exhausted, placement in a nursing center will be that much more difficult. The choices of facilities will be limited, as it will mean applying directly for the governmental assistance program.

Moreover, nursing care in the home is fraught with its own problems. Nurses, aides, or companions may become ill themselves, necessitating replacement, which might not always be satisfactory or even available. Weather problems, car problems, and personality differences are just a few of the issues that can arise.

Often, medical equipment is needed in the home, including a hospital bed with an over-the-bed table, bedside commode, etc. This can be handled effectively and efficiently in some home settings, but not all. People with substantial means can choose to do whatever they wish. Whatever the toll, if keeping Mom, Dad, or spouse at home is to be done at "all costs," that may be exactly what it will take. Just make sure that the toll doesn't include the caregiver's health.

Evelyn and her family chose to hire a full-time live-in companion to care for Grandmother when her confusion made living alone unsafe. Over a three-year period they were able, through an agency, to find capable women who would enhance Grandmother's daily life by providing three good meals, proper hygiene, and varied social activities. This arrangement was not without its problems. While on duty, each companion required almost daily assistance from Evelyn, especially when Grandmother became upset (which was often). During the companion's time off, Evelyn, her husband, her teenaged son, the cleaning woman (an absolute gem!), and

Grandmother's out-of-town daughter filled in like jigsaw puzzle pieces to make the picture whole.

After Grandmother wandered away from her apartment and was missing for seven hours one cold, rainy November day, the companion declared it was time for a change. "Evelyn, there are five of us caring for Grandmother. We are all worn out and not doing the best job. It is time for nursing home placement." Although Evelyn hated to admit it, she knew the companion was right.

At that time (late 1960s), there were very few nursing facilities in the area and most of them were not equipped to take care of wandering dementia patients. Evelyn finally found a new facility that agreed to accept Grandmother, knowing that she wandered.

The companion agreed to be the one to escort Grandmother to the nursing center so she would not connect Evelyn to the move. The family was afraid Grandmother would resent the placement, blame Evelyn, and that it would harm their close relationship.

They need not have worried. Grandmother settled in quickly, made two good friends (with mild dementia), and thought she was in a motel. Every day, she would go to the front desk and ask if she could stay another night. The woman in charge would pretend to study her charts and then with a smile, tell Grandmother that not only could she stay another night, but also that she could keep the same room.

> **TIP:** *Location is one important factor to consider when choosing a nursing or assisted living facility. Grandmother was in the only appropriate nursing facility available, but it was eight miles from home and convenient to nothing. A visit could not be combined with any other task or errand. Each visit was a separate trip. If we have a choice between two or more equally acceptable facilities, we should choose the one easier to visit.*

HOSPITAL CARE

One bit of extra advice we are going to insert here involves a different form of institution—hospitals. If our loved one with dementia is ever hospitalized, that is a time when family and friends can be very helpful. It is important that someone stay in the room with the patient at all times, if possible. After a surgical procedure, even elderly patients who do not exhibit signs of dementia are at risk for becoming temporarily confused. People with dementing illnesses become even more confused and disoriented when in strange surroundings, and that is when accidents can occur. Tripping over an IV line while going back and forth to the bathroom, falling, or becoming frightened and depressed are just a few of the things that can happen. Hospitals are no longer adequately staffed; aides are not standing around, waiting to help someone who presses a call button. Moreover, our confused loved one might not even know what the call button is, where it is, or how to use it. The hospital is a prime place for "sundowning" to happen. (We define the word *sundowning* in the appendix.)

Remember, our loved one is in a strange environment. Also, if anesthesia is involved, patients even without dementia can emerge from anesthesia worse than when they went under. Delirium (a temporary state of confusion, restlessness, and possible hallucinations), can result, and can take time to diminish.

Bottom line: we should have someone in the hospital room with our loved one 24/7 if at all possible. If there are not enough family members and friends to fill in the shifts, hire a sitter/companion from a nurses' registry. (The hospital social worker will have a list.) It will be one of the best things we ever do for our loved one and will be money well spent. Caveat: Don't feel guilty if you cannot achieve perfection in this matter.

Congratulations to readers who have traversed this chapter without automatically putting up barriers. When we bring things we fear into the light, it often allays our fears. We have tried to provide the basic information on the types of facilities available to assist in the care of our frail, elderly loved ones with Alzheimer's disease. We have also attempted to advise on ways to assess the need for placement and on ways to approach our loved ones with the idea. "Love in action" sometimes means making difficult decisions that are in our loved one's best interest. These decisions can trigger feelings of sadness and grief that need to be felt, worked through, and let go. If we repress our feelings, we pay for it later. Feelings can't go away unless they are given attention.

This chapter has just touched on a very complex subject. We have tried to present information as clearly and concisely as possible. Additional research is not only advisable, but also will be necessary if placement becomes a reality. Each state has its own criteria for financial approval for Medicaid waivers. Costs of the facilities can vary from state to state.

To any reader who may pick out this chapter exclusively to obtain information about various types of nursing care settings, we urge you not to stop with this chapter. Please also read chapters 3, 4, and 9 for additional information on family conferences and caring for the caregiver. We know what it is like to feel overwhelmed with responsibility and grief. Remember, we authors have walked the walk and are here to support you.

POSITIVE ASPECTS OF ASSISTED LIVING OR NURSING CENTER PLACEMENT

We must keep in mind the many positive aspects of assisted living or nursing center placement. Now all of the time we spend with our loved one will be quality time. We no longer have to perform the duties that upset him, evoking resentment or anger. Someone else cuts fingernails, gives baths, dispenses medicines (fill in any procedure your loved one disliked and protested). We are now the agents of happy activities. We can truly focus on what our loved ones *can* do rather than being dismayed over what they can no longer do.

We are still the primary caregiver; but now, because we are receiving adequate sleep, we can fulfill the responsibilities with a good measure of patience, perspective, and humor. As we get to know the aides and nurses in charge of our family member's care, we begin to work together as a team. We know that in any medical emergency, care is readily available.

It will take time to adjust to this station on our Alzheimer's journey. We need to be patient with ourselves and our loved ones as this adjustment takes place. Our loved ones will be aware of our demeanor. Remember, we are the safety factor in their lives. For that reason, they need to see us reacting in a positive, cheerful manner during the "settling in" phase of the journey.

As the song reminds us, we should "put on a happy face." We know how difficult this can be. We also know what a positive effect it will have on our loved one and our new care partners.

Chapter Eleven

"We Reach Acceptance"
With Love, Tears, and Humor

**Hope is the thing with feathers
That perches in the soul,
And sings the tune without the words,
And never stops at all.**

—Emily Dickinson

Throughout this book, we have used the term *Alzheimer's journey*. It is an apt metaphor. We are on a journey to places we have never been. Our maps and tour books are found in the knowledge of the disease. Our tour guides include doctors and lawyers, support-group members, daycare professionals, home health workers, and the people who answer the Helpline at the local Alzheimer's Association chapter. We need to share this journey with family members and friends. We must not travel alone.

This is a journey of life that we are taking with someone who needs our love and care. We become "care partners." For each of us, the journey differs according to the progression of the disease, the lifestyle of the travelers, and the particular family dynamics. However, the stations along the way are similar and we are all subject to some form of denial as we approach one (or many) of these stations.

We have carefully unmasked caregiver denial along the journey and have found the fear that feeds it. We discovered that we are not alone in our denial. It is a normal, natural reaction to adversity. We authors have shared our own stories, and in combination, the many stories we have heard and been a part of in our work with people dealing with AD. We hope some of these stories have resonated with your own experiences.

Throughout the chapters, we have shared ways to shed denial by moving into positive action. We have given you, the reader, valuable knowledge about the disease. We have passed on the tips, tools, and techniques that we found have helped smooth the rough places; we shared a "prescription for a healthy caregiver." On our own journeys, we have used these ideas with great success.

TWO DIFFERENT KINDS OF ACCEPTANCE

It is time, now, to talk about acceptance. We hope that you have been experiencing acceptance in small ways throughout the journey. We need to look at the big picture and see what we mean by *acceptance*. Acceptance is an attitude, a way of thinking and behaving that encompasses a given situation. Will we receive this situation, namely, Alzheimer's disease, with grace? Or will we grudgingly bear up and accept our fate? Those are two very different types of acceptance. One is accomplished through love and laughter; the other holds resentment and regret. We hope you will choose love and laughter.

Just as we have had to work our way out of denial, we need to work our way into a healthy acceptance. How can we accept a disease as difficult as Alzheimer's? There is no cure. It causes us to gradually lose the one we love—it is the "long good-bye." It demands 24/7 care. It changes our lives in ways that are not to our liking. But Alzheimer's disease is the *given*. We can't send it back. We've discovered we cannot deny its presence. It is here, a part of our lives. This fact we cannot change. We can imitate Charlie Brown and keep our head down, immersed in a cloud of despair. Or we can take Lucy's five-cent advice: "Lift up your head, Charlie Brown, and smile. You will feel better."

INGREDIENTS OF HEALTHY ACCEPTANCE

Healthy acceptance is dependent on a healthy attitude. Our attitude adjustment will take time and much practice. We need to be patient, for our progress will be uneven. There will be many days when we will want to throw in the towel. We will make mistakes. We will cry. This is all part of the fabric of acceptance. We need to be honest about our feelings and frustrations. Healthy acceptance does not require us to deny the reality of our situation; it does ask us to introduce large quantities of humor.

Steve Allen, author, musician, and TV personality of the 1950s, had this to say about humor: "Humor is the essence of humanity. The sadness of life, far from totally discouraging laughter, gives rise to it. Jokes are always about things that are wrong. We laugh at our tragedies in order to prevent our suffering."

When we Alzheimer's caregivers find humor in our daily lives, we give ourselves a precious gift. Evelyn discovered that, often, a difficult and frustrating experience would later prove humorous. The knowledge that she would laugh later made the difficult situation more bearable. "I will laugh at this tomorrow," she would tell herself. And she always did.

Ellen's mother and aunt said and did such "cute" things that she began to write them down. Her experiences with them, as well as with the patients she worked with in the hospital, became a collection and then a book, *Between Two Worlds*.

Those of us who are able to keep our sense of humor while keeping our senses as we face life's adversities are making the "hero's choice" and taking the "hero's journey." We caregivers need to seek a balance—that delicate balance between enduring a difficult situation and lightening our load through the use of humor.

Acceptance depends on our desire for it, the honest assessment of our situation, and a large dose of humor that helps us cope with our fatigue, frustrations, and sadness. But the most important ingredient in the mix of attitude enhancers and fostering healthy acceptance is love: love that is identified by action. It is love that caregivers provide from the very beginning of the journey. It is love that has held us together when we thought we might break from the heartache and sorrow of Alzheimer's disease. It is love that has held us fast to the task when we "wished to be in Cancun." It is love that shines out of our loved ones' eyes when we give them comfort and security. And most surely it is love they feel when we introduce laughter and joy into their difficult days.

OUR LOVED ONES WORK THROUGH THEIR ACCEPTANCE

Our loved ones have their own trouble accepting the Alzheimer's diagnosis. Evelyn remembers how her husband utilized his keen sense of humor so often during the early stages of the disease. One late spring day in Yosemite Valley, California, Evelyn was drinking in the view of four large waterfalls. Later in the year, they would dry up; but on that early June day they were still being fed by melting snow. Evelyn turned to her husband, John, to tell him, "I want to etch this scene onto my brain. I don't want to forget this beauty." John replied, in a tone that underscored the humor he intended, "I'll be lucky if I remember this view five minutes from now."

Our loved ones are working through their own acceptance. They may never speak about their disease, but this does not mean that they are unaware of the changes in their lives.

The following poem appeared in the Greater Maryland Chapter of the Alzheimer's Association's Newsletter in 1995. It aptly describes the plight of the person with Alzheimer's:

> Please try to understand what I am now,
> Not think of me as I once was.
> I am alone, shut in with my fears
> My frustrations, my forgetfulness.
> Forgive me if I strike out at you. Why do I do that?
> What happened to me? I cannot cope with this alien world.
> I feel threatened. I am frightened.
> Speak softly, approach slowly.
> Repeat again and again what you want of me.
> Those twisted tangles in my brain have messed up my world.
> Be patient, for I do love you, and I need your help and love
> So very, very much.
>
> —Your Alzheimer's Patient

In the early stages of the disease, John tried to help his sister, Helen, with AD, keep track of the days of the week. He showed her all the tricks he had devised to remember simple things. The notebook in his shirt pocket worked wonders until he could no longer read the written word nor write it. Even then, he kept the notebook because Evelyn would write a note on it before he left for daycare. He couldn't read the note, but he knew it was there; a tie to Evelyn and security.

After John stopped driving, he told Evelyn, "I really miss driving. I know I shouldn't drive anymore, but I don't like giving it up. I don't fuss because I can't change anything." Evelyn thought John's acceptance was better than her own.

We know that John's acceptance may not be the norm. Evelyn feels that one important factor contributing to John's behavior was his participation in an early-stage memory loss support group. For six months he was a member of this group, meeting twice a month with other people who were experiencing losses similar to his own. They shared their anger and frustrations. They shared the techniques they had devised to compensate for their memory loss. The understanding that he was not alone in his problem was comforting. John bonded with the other participants. They became a team, giving each other a sense of well-being in the midst of the catastrophic change in their lives.

Dear caregiver, if your loved one is in the early stages of the disease, try to find an early-stage support group for him or her.

ACCESSING MIRTH

After publication in 1999 of her first book, *Between Two Worlds*, Ellen, often with Evelyn's participation, gave talks and workshops on humor as the gift that keeps on giving. The talks were usually titled "VITAMIN H—Humor for Care-givers" or "VITAMIN H—The Humor Treatment." The catch phrase that Ellen coined and used throughout the book was *access mirth*. She felt that caregivers with smiles on their faces enhanced both their own lives and the lives of their loved ones with Alzheimer's. Smiles can lower the anxiety level of our loved ones. They absorb our mood. How much better for us, and for them, if we can foster a sense of peace and comfort rather than fear and "dis-ease."

A smile, even if forced, makes us feel better (try it now). We should not wait for an external event to make us smile. Smile first, and we find that our attitude toward our situation will change. We don't smile because we are happy; we are happy because we smile.

GRADUAL DEVELOPMENT OF HEALTHY ACCEPTANCE

Healthy acceptance is developed gradually as we learn to deal with each station on our Alzheimer's journey. Some stages of the disease are harder than others to accept. Evelyn found her husband's language loss to be a devastating development. She relates, "After I finally 'chewed that up and swallowed it,' other losses were easier to accept."

Acceptance means we can admit that we don't like what's happening, that we can cry. But it also means we will make that effort to dry the tears and find a smile. Acceptance does not solve all the problems; it makes them easier to live with. It helps us to say, "Things will never be the same again," and understand that we can find in our new lives a good measure of love, joy, and happiness.

We will join with other caregivers who have walked the road from denial through anger to action and acceptance, over and over again, and declare:

- I will move forward and deal with life one day at a time (sometimes one hour at a time).
- I will be grateful for every patch of blue sky.
- I will make the most of the hand I have been dealt.
- I will smile and laugh along the way. My loved one needs to see a smile on my face, not a frown.
- I will seek information.
- I will seek help in a support group.
- I will look for beauty in my everyday life.
- I will grieve, for I am losing my loved one.
- I will cry.
- I will love.
- I will heal.

APPENDIX

Activities of Daily Living (ADLs)
Dressing
Hygiene (bathing, etc.)
Feeding
Toileting (bladder and bowel control)
Mobility (The ability to get in and out of a bed or chair. If in a wheelchair, the ability to transfer to and from a bed or chair.)

The Four As
Amnesia—The partial or total loss of memory.
Aphasia—A total or partial loss of the power to use or understand words.
Agnosia—The inability to recognize something as what it is, e.g., the sound of a doorbell, the smell of something burning, the look of a piece of clothing, the use of an eating utensil.
Apraxia—Complete or partial loss of memory of how to perform complex muscular movements, resulting from damage to certain areas of the brain. For example, getting out of a chair, a bed, or even walking may be unachievable.

Functions of Daily Living
Shopping
Cooking
Using the telephone
Light housekeeping
Keeping track of simple finances
Arranging for necessary transportation

175

Legal Matters

Durable Power of Attorney

The durable power of attorney document is the tool that allows the person with dementia to designate a trusted friend or family member to carry out all financial decisions when the person with dementia is no longer deemed competent. These decisions must be consistent with the best interests of the person with dementia. It is the term *durable* that makes the document valid when the person is no longer competent.

The power of attorney for the healthcare documents allows the person with dementia to designate a trusted friend or family member to make all the healthcare decisions when the person is no longer able.

Living Will, or Advance Directive

In this document the person with dementia states his wishes concerning artificial life-support when a doctor deems that the person is terminally ill.

Sundowning

A term used to describe the confused, agitated, pacing behaviors that may occur late in the day "after the sun goes down." It may continue into the evening, causing a disruption in the sleep pattern. This behavior is common with AD patients who are hospitalized. The cause is unknown. It may be related to the biological clock in the brain, the fatigue of the patient, or the changes in light patterns.

RESOURCE MATERIAL AVAILABLE FROM THE ALZHEIMER'S ASSOCIATION

Brochures
Activities at Home
Alzheimer's Disease: The Basics
Behaviors
Caregiver Stress
Communication

Helpline 24/7
If You Have Alzheimer's Disease
Late-stage Care
Legal Plans
Living with Early-onset Alzheimer's Disease
Living with Early-stage Alzheimer's Disease
Money Matters
Personal Care
Safe at Home
Safe Return
Ten Warning Signs

Fact Sheets

Adult Daycare
Alzheimer's Disease
Bathing
Depression and Alzheimer's Disease
Dressing
Driving
Eating
Feelings
Grief, Mourning, Guilt
Holidays
Hospitalization
Incontinence
Sexuality
Sleep Changes in Alzheimer's Disease
Telling the Person, Family and Friends
Vacationing

For a complete list of fact sheets, go to http://www.alz.org/Resources/ Factsheets.asp

Hotlines and Web Sites

- Alzheimer's Association
  Phone: 1-800-272-3900
  E-mail: info@alz.org
  Web site: http://www.alz.org

- Alzheimer's Association Helpline
  Phone: 1-800-443-2273 (This is answered 24/7.)

- Safe Return
  Phone: 1-888-572-8566
  Web site: http://www.alz.org/safereturn

The Alzheimer's Association's Safe Return program helps reunite persons with dementia who have wandered away from their family members and/or caregivers. 24/7 assistance is provided.

Library

Green-Field Library: The Alzheimer's Association Green-Field Library is the nation's largest Alzheimer's library. The library offers many information services to the public. Information about the library, its services, and the online catalog can be found at http://www.alz.org/Services/Library/Services.asp.

Message Boards and Chat Rooms

Log on to the 24/7 online support community for people with Alzheimer's, family caregivers, and professional caregivers at:
    http://www.alz.org/messageboards
    Browse messages anonymously. No sign-up required. No personal data captured.

Videos

Check with your local Alzheimer's Association chapter as to availability of the following tapes. Or check online at http://www.alz.org/Resources/Resources/rtrlcorelist.asp.

Alzheimer's Disease: At Time of Diagnosis. Glenwood, IA: Info Vision, 1996.
Alzheimer's Disease: Inside Looking Out. Chicago: Terra Nova Films, 1995.
Alzheimer's Journey. Toronto: Alzheimer Society of Canada, 1998.
Beloved Strangers: Caring for a Loved One with Alzheimer's Disease. Medfield, MA: Aquarius Health Care Videos, 2003.
Best friends. Chicago: Terra Nova Films, 1993.
Caring about Howard. Durham, NC: Educational Media Services, 1998.
Complaints of a Dutiful Daughter. New York: Women Make Movies, 1994.
Coping with Alzheimer's: You Are Not Alone. Madison: University of Wisconsin Extension Publications, 1995.
Diagnosis and Management of Persons with Dementia. Los Angeles: Alzheimer's Association, Los Angeles Chapter, 1998.
Early-onset Memory Loss: A Conversation with Letty Tennis. Chicago: Terra Nova Films, 1992.
Facing Alzheimer's: An African-American Perspective. Northfield, IL: TMK Productions, 2002.
The Forgetting. St. Paul, MN: Twin Cities Public Television, 2003.
From Here to Hope. Durham, NC: Educational Media Services, 1998.
How to Communicate Effectively with Someone Who Has Alzheimer's Disease. Medford, OR: Healing Arts Communications, 2001.
Living in Alzheimer's Disease. San Diego: George G. Glenner Alzheimer's Family Centers, 1999.
Prescription for Caregivers: Take Care of Yourself. Chicago: Terra Nova Films, 1995.
Sundowning: A Caregiver's Guide. San Marcos, CA: Advanced Healthcare Studies, 2003.

SUGGESTED READING

Alterra, Aaron. *The Caregiver: A Life with Alzheimer's*. South Royalton, VT: Steerforth Press, 1999. Testimonials by John Bayley and Reeve Lindberg.

Bell, Virginia, and David Troxel. *The Best Friends Approach to Alzheimer's Care*. London, Winnipeg, Sydney: Health Professions Press, 1997. This book shows how easily you can make a difference in the life of a family member or a client in your care.

Burger, Sarah Green, Virginia Fraser, Sara Hunt, and Barbara Frank. *Nursing Homes: Getting Good Care There*. 2nd ed. Atascadero, CA: Impact Publishers, 2002. You want the best possible care for your loved one who lives in a nursing home. An essential resource for caring families and patient advocates, this consumer action guide will help you get it.

Coste, Joanne Koenig. *Learning to Speak Alzheimer's: A Groundbreaking Approach for Everyone Dealing with the Disease*. Boston: Houghton Mifflin, 2003. Coste offers a practical approach to the emotional well-being of both caregivers and their loved ones with AD. It emphasizes relating to persons with AD in their own reality.

Dunn, Hank. *Hard Choices for Loving People: CPR, Artificial Feeding, Comfort Care and the Patient with a Life-Threatening Illness*. 4th ed. Herndon, VA: A & A Publishers, 2000.

Ewing, Wayne. *Tears in God's Bottle: Reflections on Alzheimer's Caregiving*. Tucson, AZ: Whitestone Circle Press, 1999. A series of groundbreaking reflections chronicling the author's struggle with his jumbled emotions of love, loss, sorrow, quiet anger, selfishness, and hope. This book offers insight and sustenance drawn from the Old Testament and the New Testament.

Feil, Naomi, and Vicki DeKlerk-Rubino. *The Validation Breakthrough: Simple Techniques for Communicating with People with "Alzheimer's Type" Dementia*. Baltimore: Health Professions Press, 1996.

Gordon, Barry. *Remembering and Forgetting in Everyday Life*. Baltimore: Mastermedia, 1995.

Haisman, Pam. *Alzheimer's Disease: Caregivers Speak Out*. Fort Myers, FL: Chippendale House Publishers, 1998.

Manning, Doug. *When Love Gets Tough: The Nursing Home Decision*. Hereford, TX: In-Sight Books, 1983. A warm, wonderful booklet that goes step-by-step through the placement process.

McGowin, Diana Friel. *Living in the Labyrinth: A Personal Journal through the Maze of Alzheimer's Disease*. New York: Delta, 1994.

Murphy, Beverly Bigtree. *He Used to Be Somebody: A Journey into Alzheimer's Disease through the Eyes of a Caregiver*. Boulder, CO: Gibbs Associates, 1995.

Rabins, Peter, and Nancy L. Mace. *The 36-Hour Day*. 3rd ed. Baltimore: Johns Hopkins University Press, 1999.

Radin, Lisa, and Gary Radin, eds. *What If It's Not Alzheimer's? A Caregiver's Guide to Dementia*. Amherst, NY: Prometheus Books, 2003.

Robinson, Anne, Beth Spencer, and Laurie White. *Understanding Difficult Behaviors: Some Practical Suggestions for Coping with Alzheimer's Disease and Related Illnesses*. Ypsilanti: Eastern Michigan University, 2002. First published in 1991.

Warner, Mark. *The Complete Guide to Alzheimer's-Proofing Your Home*. West Lafayette, IN: Purdue University Press, 1998.

Young, Ellen. *Between Two Worlds: Special Moments of Alzheimer's and Dementia*. Amherst, NY: Prometheus Books, 1999.

REMEMBER: There is always help available, 24/7, at the Alzheimer's Association Helpline: 1-800-443-2273